# LIVE One Hour
# YOGA Sessions

Dipanshu Aggarwal

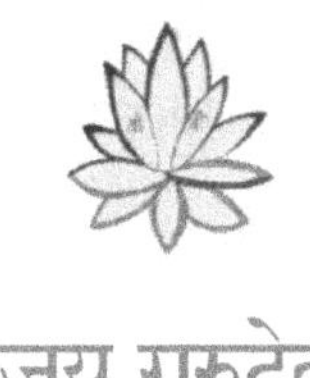

जय गुरुदेव

Title: **Live One Hour Yoga Sessions**
Author: **Dipanshu Aggarwal**

Printed and Published by
**Devotees of Sri Sri Ravi Shankar Ashram**
34 Sunny Enclave, Devigarh Road,
Patiala 147001, Punjab, India

https://advaita56.weebly.com/
The Art of Living Centre

https://www.artofliving.org/

18th December 2021 Narayana Poornima, Dattatreya Jayanti
Rohini Nakshatra, Bhadra, Sarvartha Siddhi Yoga, Margashirsha
Vikram Samvat 2078 Ananda, Saka Era 1943 Plava

1st Edition December 2021

जय गुरुदेव

# Dedication

## Sri Sri Ravi Shankar

who revealed to us the powerful breathing technique known as the
**Sudarshan Kriya**

**an offering at thy lotus feet**

## Front Cover Image Credits

Dipanshu on the Yoga Mat demonstrating Warrior II =
*Virabhadrāsana* Posture. Date 20 Feb 2021 10:06am.


Images within the book courtesy morning Yoga Session 5:45am 21
July 2021 by Dipanshu.

# Acknowledgements

Grateful thanks to all who attend yoga sessions in my Yoga Studio. Some mentions:

*sangeeta seema ashish urmila somnath aparna*

*seema ashish urmila somnath aparna*

*ashish urmila somnath aparna*

*urmila somnath aparna*

*somnath aparna*

*pavani*

*somnath aparna*

*urmila somnath aparna*

*ashish urmila somnath aparna*

*seema ashish urmila somnath aparna*

*sangeeta seema ashish urmila somnath aparna*

# Blessing

All in all, Yoga is such a boon to mankind that nobody should be deprived of it. Because everyone has the right to peace, everyone has the right to be in deep love and everyone has the right to be healthy.

Make sure to let this goodness of Yoga reach to every doorstep. Yoga is the best tool for us to blossom in human values. It can help us to get rid of stress, physical fatigue, emotional turbulence, and will bring mental clarity.

Sri Sri Ravi Shankar
International Day of Yoga, June 21, 2021

# Prayer

योगेन चित्तस्य पदेन वाचां मलं शरीरस्य च वैद्यकेन ।

योऽपाकरोत्तं प्रवरं मुनीनां पतञ्जलिं प्राञ्जलिरानतोऽस्मि ॥

yogena cittasya padena vācāṃ malaṃ śarīrasya ca vaidyakena |

yo'pākarottaṃ pravaraṃ munīnāṃ patañjaliṃ prāñjalirānato'smi ||


To the revered sage Patanjali, who gave us
        by Yogic practice the purity of Mind,
        by Grammar the sweetness of Tongue,
        by Ayurveda a cure for illness of Body,
to him my heartfelt salutation.

# Contents

# Preface

The one of the few things that I am certain of, from my experiences, studies and contemplations, is that a good rest is of paramount importance to live a fulfilling life. But, today, the world has become so capitalist that we look not for a good rest but for a productive rest. Our desire for gain drives *how* we rest – we want to grow hair, get rid of spinal misalignments, or improve digestion while we are sleeping. It is ironic, since a good rest first demands not a relaxed body, but a relaxed mind.

I do not have any illusions regarding my capabilities regarding convincing people to lose this way of thinking. Hence, I wish to contribute to provide productive rest but with one change – a productive rest what will also relax the mental and the emotional body – resulting in true rest that is found in deep silence. I know this to be achievable by Yoga, and that I wholeheartedly endorse.

Time is of the essence – hence the need for productive rest. While we cannot increase the number of hours given to us, we can surely increase the efficiency and quality of the time we utilize. From this thought has sprung the idea of writing a book that gives sequence of asanas and other yogic elements that can be practiced in under 1 hour.

Today, most of us have poor posture. There is so much one can do to sit straight – it seems quite impossible to have a perfect posture. Poor posture severely and primarily affects the spine, which controls the brain health and mental clarity. The other major areas that are affected are the shoulders and the hips. The other aspect that is affected is the digestion process. A poor digestive system affects the emotional health – and emotions collect in our shoulders and hips, making them stiffer.

A stiff body, a dull mind, and unstable emotions are in no way conducive for good sleep – and the system starts to crash. Many of us have become accustomed to this quality of life that we are not even aware what a good healthy body-mind matrix feels like.

Yogic asana and pranayama have been developed in such a way that they work on multiple aspects at once. The asanas realign the muscles of the body to their correct position, improve digestion and the hormonal balance.

The breath and our attention to the breath and body remove the mental dullness and the emotional toxicity that collects in the body and mind. Once the body is in a good state while awake, it is active, productive and lively. Consequently, a day well spent leads to a night well rested – sleep automatically becomes deep and peaceful and rhythmic.

I hope you can find some value from this book.

# Diet

Bhagavad Gita

युक्ताहारविहारस्य युक्तचेष्टस्य कर्मसु । युक्तस्वभावबोधस्य योगो भवति दुःखहा ॥ ६.१७

yuktaahaaravihaarasya, yuktace.s.tasya karmasu ।

yuktasvapnaavabodhasya, yogo bhavati du.hkhahaa ॥ 6.17

6.17 Be regulated in food and exercise; be balanced in activity and duty. Take proper sleep and rest, and nurture senses equitably. Such a lifestyle leads to freedom from pain. It frees one from suffering. It extinguishes the pangs of remorse and banishes turmoil from life.

# Pranayama

Patanjali Yoga Sutra

ततः क्षीयते प्रकाशावरणम् ॥ ५२ ॥ tataḥ kṣīyate prakāśāvaraṇam

**2.52 Then the veil on the Divinity within becomes shorn.**
Regular practice of Pranayama removes the emotional thought web and painful memory cladding from the Soul. When learnt properly from a Master and practiced sincerely, pranayama uncovers the mask that obscures the purity within us.

- Ujjayi Breath – "snoring" breath with focus on throat muscles. Sound of breath touching throat is clearly audible.
- Kapal Bhati – forceful breath expulsion with focus on the navel, the incoming breath is natural.
- Bhastrika – forceful noisy breath, like a piston.
- Brahmari – meditative breathing with humming bee sound from closed lips.
- Nadi Shodhan – alternate nostril breathing, with focus on the nose. Silent, calm and normal breathing.

# Meditation

## Patanjali Yoga Sutra

ध्यानहेयास्तद्वृत्तयः ॥ ११ ॥ dhyānaheyāstadvṛttayaḥ

**2.11 Meditation shall alleviate such thoughts.**

Meditation will help erase troublesome thoughts and memories. It will remove the mind-conditioning due to stress, trauma, pain and fear.

Meditation is the best "soap" for making the mind clear and the heart soft. It helps one to function to the best of one's ability and live a cheerful compassionate life.

# Essentials

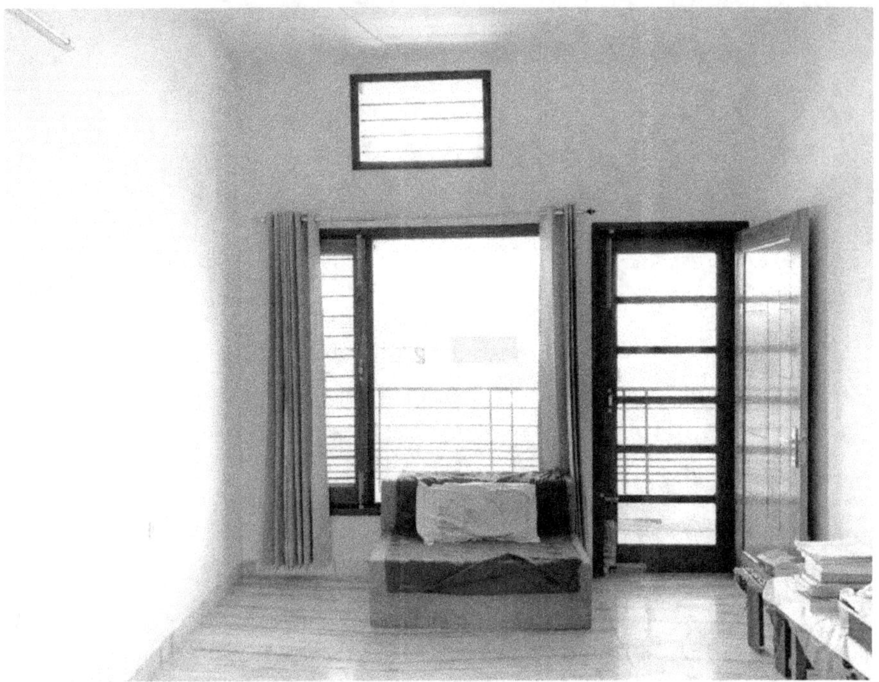

Well-Ventilated and Lighted Room with enough clear space.

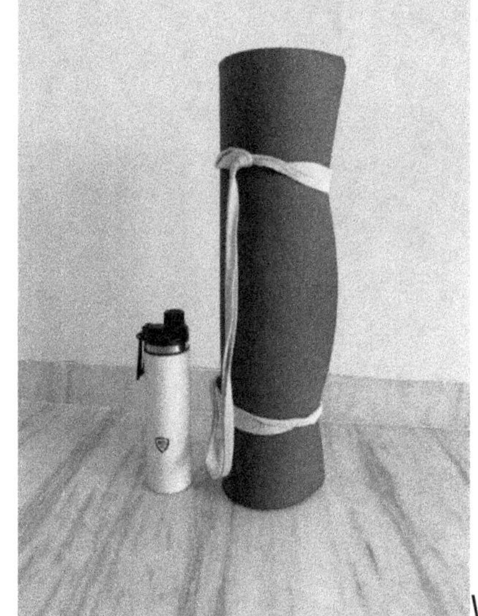

Water Bottle, Yoga Mat

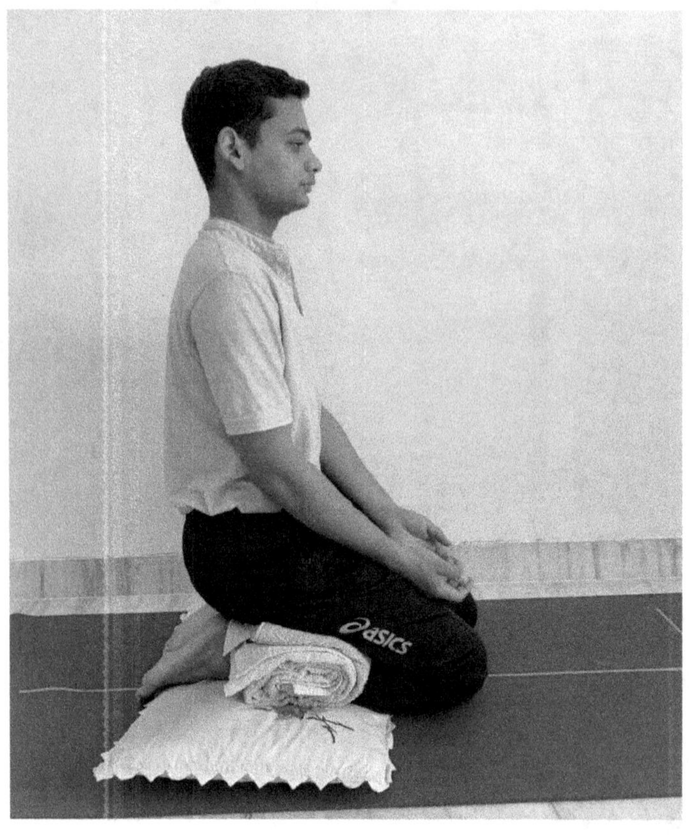

Demonstration of Yoga Knee Cushion

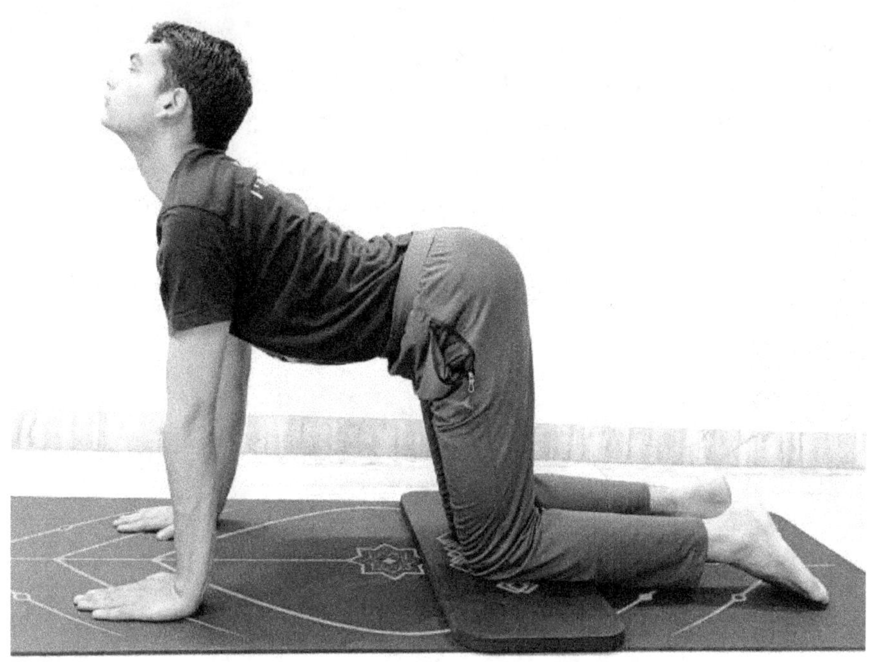

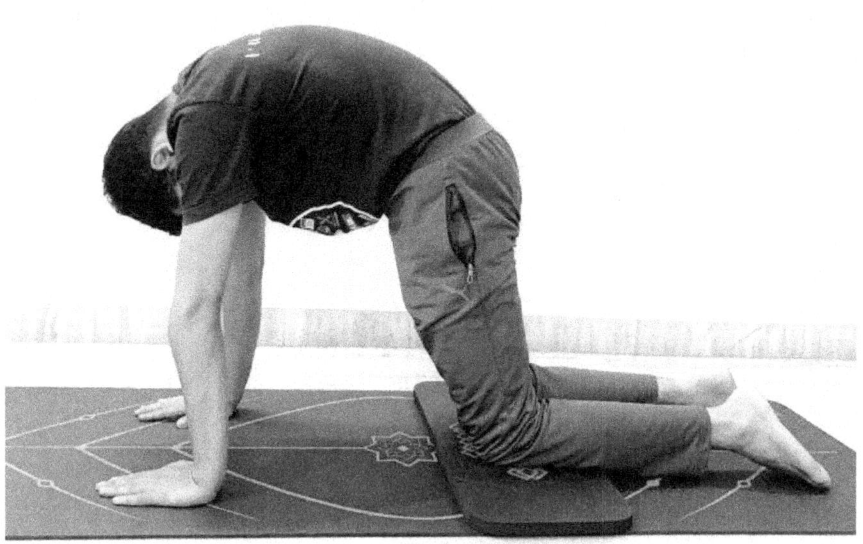

# Asana flow during 1 Hour Session

### Prelude
Go out for a brisk walk of a KM for twenty minutes. Spend some time in nature with the sun, birds, leaves. Observe the sky, become friends with nature, flora and fauna, the small animals you see. Please do keep your smartphone and wallet at home during the walk and nature time. Please ensure you are not carrying or wearing any electronic gadgets. Yoga is not for the faint hearted.

### Room Readiness
Ensure proper ventilation, warmth, lighting in the room. Take out your Yoga Mat. See that it is clean, not dusty nor soiled. Use a good quality mat.

Keep a bolster, rolled up towel, and a pillow and cushion handy. Keep your smartphone and gadgets out of hearing, out of sight and out of mind.

This is not a zoom session, this ain't an online class. You shall not be hearing any music nor fiddling with the volume or viewing angle, not watching any TV or youtube drill. This is an inward journey, where your senses, intellect, memory shall get aligned and tuned to your breath and body. To yourself, to the Being that is you.

## Warm up with close attention to Body and Breath
Warm up and making yourself comfortable by some body massage, stretching and joint movement. Do as you like, be it dance or slow swaying or massage. Bring attention to your body. Notice that feet muscles are loose, ankle joints are moving freely, and shoulders are relaxed. Close the eyes and take a deep breath in. Relax your neck as you breath out. Take another breath in and bring your attention to the chest. Keep your abdomen a little tight, so that you are breathing from the chest and not from the abdomen. Feel your chest expand and contract with every inhalation and exhalation. Observe your breath with attention on the chest. Breath with a rhythm, just like soft music. Continue for a couple of minutes with awareness. Another deep breath in, hold the breath for a few seconds, and then exhale completely, exhale the last drop. Another breath in, move your attention to the heart. Notice any sensations at the heart.

## OM Chant or a short Prayer of your choice
We shall chant OM thrice. Breathe in for Om, and upon exhalation chant long, loud, and clear. With each breath make the Om chant modulated, clearer and longer. Hear your chant, and be aware of the sensations in the region of your heart. Make each breath deeper, smoother, steadier, keeping full awareness.

Relax and be silent for a couple of minutes, hear the silence.


## Pranayama with Forceful Breaths
We shall begin with Bhastrika Pranayama. Make sure you are comfortable in the posture, if needed use a rolled-up towel under your hips or a pillow under the ankles. Sit on a mat, bedroll or a blanket. Sit straight, with a smile and a cheerful countenance.

Sit in Vajrasana, get in position for the first round of bhastrika, loose fists at shoulder level, nails pointing to front, thumbs outside. During each forceful inhalation, the hands are thrown vertically and get maximum straight stretched, the fists open palms wide. During each forceful exhalation, the hands drop to shoulder level, fists close. Do this to a count of 20 breaths. Relax with open palms on knees facing the sky for few seconds. Notice the flow of energy in the limbs and torso.  Repeat for 3 rounds of 20 breaths each, with alert relaxation after each round.

Now come out of Vajrasana. Stretch and massage the hands and legs and knees. Pat the calves. Sit comfortably in sukhasana.

CLOCK 11 minutes elapsed
**Pelvic Rotations**
Sit comfortably. Cross-legged posture. Lock your palms on your knees. Breathe in, drop your head back, push your chest towards the sky. After a moment, as you exhale bend forward, take your head to the floor. Touch your forehead to the ground and stay there a moment.

Breathe in, move to the right, start sitting body rotation. Keep your eyes closed and focus on the movement. Make full clockwise circles, taking conscious breaths. Keep the face relaxed.

At the half circle as your body goes back, exhale, and at the complete circle as your torso comes fore, inhale. Maintain a comfortable pace, stretch your torso in wide circles, synchronize your breathing with the half circles.

At the end of six clockwise circles, touch your forehead to the ground and stay there a moment.

Now slowly begin the other way (anticlockwise). Gradually increase pace to be in a comfortable rhythm. Stretch torso full out in large circles. Synchronize breath and rotation.

If the body has any urges…belching, sneezing, coughing…stop a while, release your urges, and then continue.

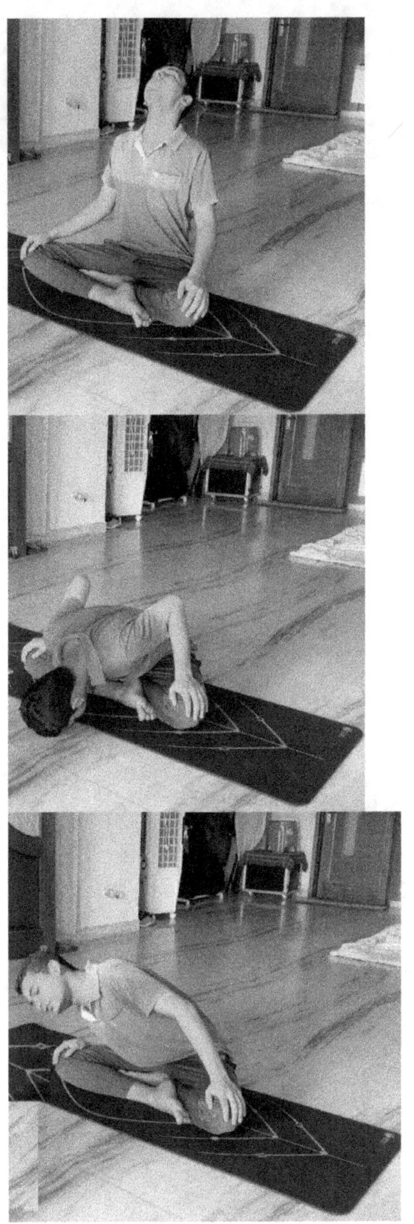

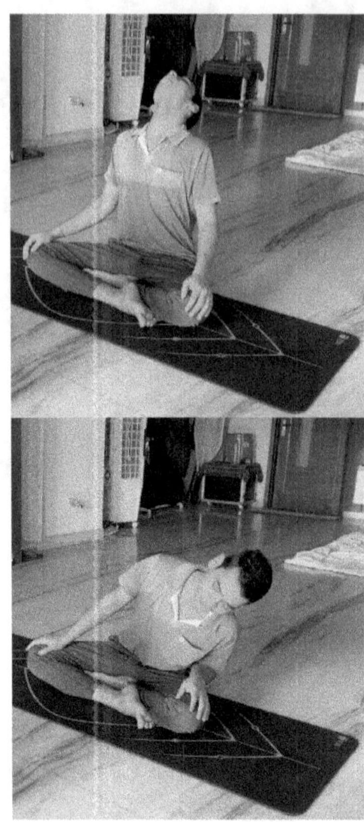

Do six rounds anti clockwise body rotation, at the end allow the forehead to touch the ground. Stay there a moment, and breathe in and come up and tilt back all the way. Push your jaws to the sky, let your throat pull your chest up. Stay there a moment.

Engage the pelvic floor, contract, lift it up.
Engage the navel, pull it in. Drop your head back a little more.
Inhale, hold the breath in, bring your neck to touch the chest, holding the contractions of the pelvis and the nabhi.

Push the knees down, straighten your elbows, make the arms taut. Straighten the head.  Exhale slowly, releasing the contractions. Open the eyes, massage the thighs and knees.

### Bandha Locks
Sit with the abdomen engaged. As you breathe in, tighten the anus muscles, and take the head back. Then hold the breath and lower

your neck and bring it to the chest. Hold for a few seconds such that you are comfortable, then gently release the neck and exhale and release the anus muscles.

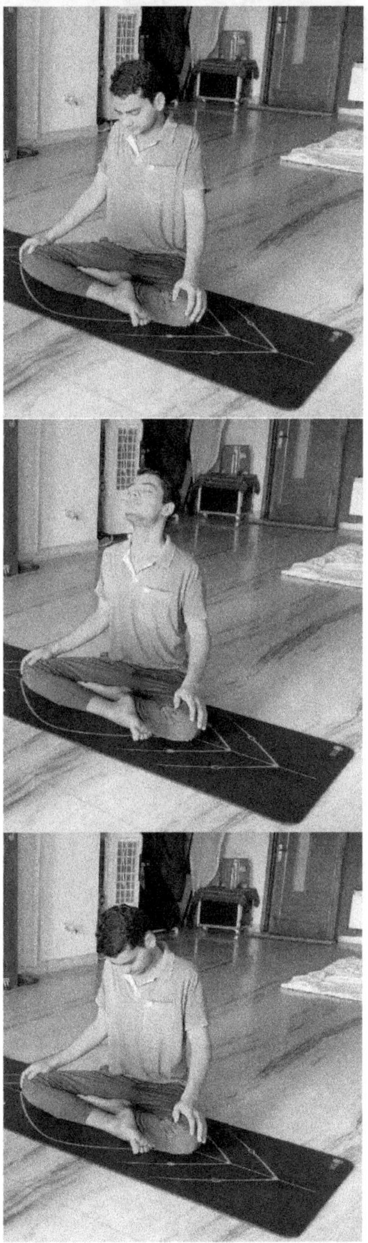

**Arm Movements**

Sit comfortably in sukhasana. Start shaking your hands. Move your arms all around, up and down like falling rain, like a gush of wind. Any way you like, make circles, remember it is only arm movements, torso and head steady. Give your arms a good shake. Increase the speed slowly, go all out, uninhibited.

Keep moving, flailing, for a couple of minutes. Gradually decrease the speed and stop. Be with yourself for a moment, observe the sensations in the body, let the breath become normal.

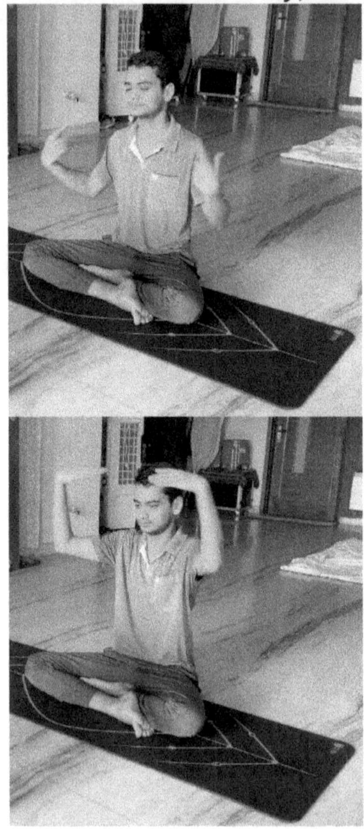

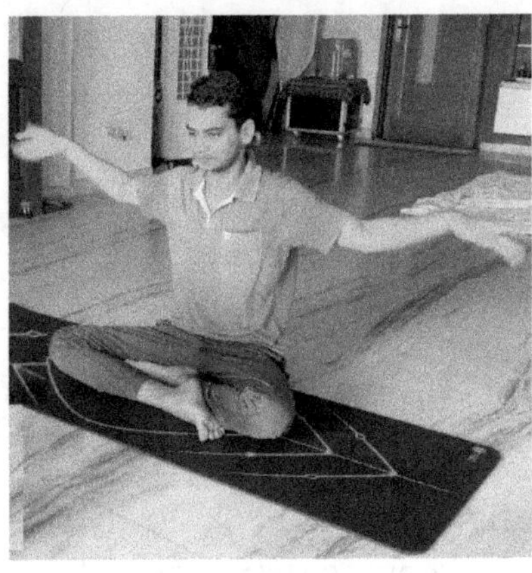

CLOCK 16 minutes elapsed
**Jogging with Arm Shoulder Elbow Wrist Finger Movements (Freestyle Dance)**
Slowly stand up, and start jogging in place. Keep your attention on your limbs. Shoulders loose. Move around a bit, and jog with awareness. Start pumping shoulders, flex your wrists and fingers.

If the mind starts remembering and planning and nudging…office, dinner, picnic…erase all that, bring the attention back to the body, and continue.

Lift your arms up, continue jogging. Shuffle sideways. Shuffle back and forth. Jump up and down. Legs to the front, legs to the back, knees to the palms, twists, dances, whoops.

Continue for three minutes, increasing the pace to the maximum for the final jog, then slow down and become still.

Stand still. Stand in silence. Honor yourself. Honor your body. Honor your mind. Be grateful for this creation and this planet. Allow your breath to become normal.

If the body has any urges…belching, sneezing, coughing…stop a while, release your urges.

CLOCK 19minutes elapsed
Hum sound for easing out emotions and blocks in the chest and navel.

From a standing posture, breathe in and bend back slowly all the way, raising and extending your arms, keeping them parallel. Keep the feet firmly grounded. Now breathe in and bend forward and down, flailing the arms all the way and saying "Hum" loudly. Repeat thrice.

CLOCK 21 minutes elapsed
**Back, Side and Front Bends for Spinal Strength and Alignment**

From a standing straight posture, breathe in and go back slowly all the way, raising and extending your arms, keeping them parallel. Keep the feet firmly grounded. Legs steady. Stay in the posture for six good breaths, then with an exhalation come back to a straight posture. Drop your arms.

From a standing straight posture, breathe in and raise the right arm vertical, slowly twist the neck and tilt the head to look at the right palm. Allow your left hand to slide along the thigh and be taut. Stay in the posture for six good breaths, then with an exhalation come back to a straight posture. Arms to the sides loose.

Repeat on the other side, with the left hand vertical on top and the right hand taut on the thigh.

From a standing straight posture, inhale and raise both arms parallel and vertical over the head. Feel a full stretch all the way in the body. Steady the legs, and with as you exhale, do a "Hum" sound, bend forward and let your arms swing down towards your knees. Inhale and straighten up. Adjust your feet and legs, adjust your shoulders and wrists, become calm.

Abdomen tight, pulled in, hips engaged. Repeat thrice with an instantaneous "Hum" emanating from the throat region. Then stand still, silent, grateful.

Observe the senses, eyes, ears, mouth...Become aware of their immense use and potential to do good for the planet, and for YOU.

**Triangle, Warrior Poses, Enhance the Courage, Assertiveness, Principles**

From a standing straight posture, stretch your legs wide, three feet apart. Move the right foot to be at 90° and adjust the left foot to be at 10° relative to the torso. Upper body is facing the front wall. Breathe in, arms go up to shoulder level, palms outstretched on either side. Breathe out, reach out to the right side, bending at the waist, as if you are trying to reach someone to your right. Knees are straight, there is no knee bend here.

Breathe in and breathe out, right hand goes down towards the right ankle, left hand reaches for the sky. Feel the right bend at the waist, without any twist nor any forward dropping. Turn your neck to look up at the left palm. Steady the weight on your legs and feet. Maintain the posture for six good breaths.

Breathe in and breathe out, right arm comes up and right elbow placed on right knee, left arm moves from vertical to angle over the head to the right. Left arm to the left leg is one straight line. See there is a spring in the body as you go deep in the stretch.

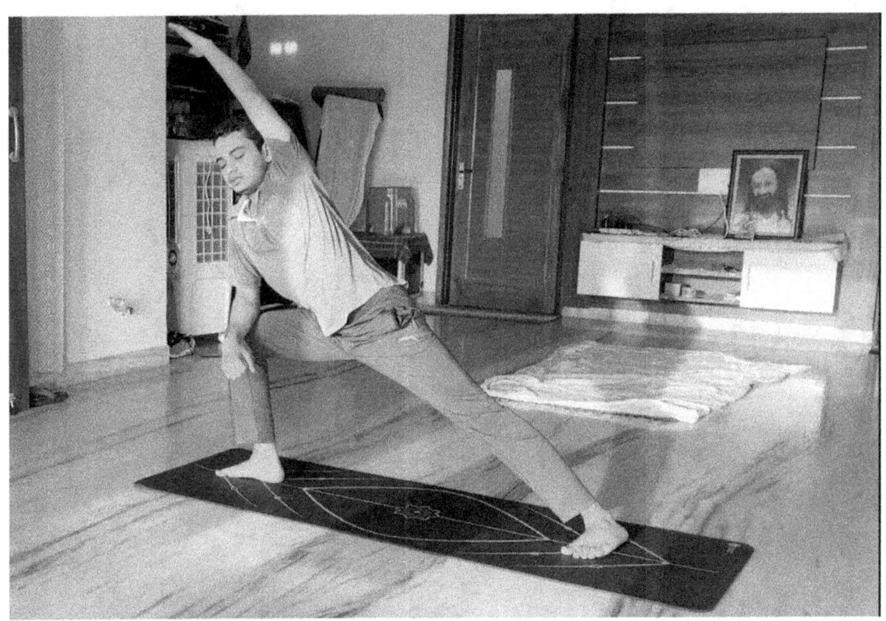

Breathe in and breathe out, left arm lowers to touch the left thigh, right knee straightens as you come out of the posture and stand with arms to the sides.

Become stable and steady, legs and feet are still outstretched.

We shall repeat this pose on the other side.

Gently rotate the right foot and the left foot so that the left foot is now  at 90° and the right foot is at 10° relative to the torso. Notice there is no forward bend. Slowly repeat the entire set on this side.

Warrior 1

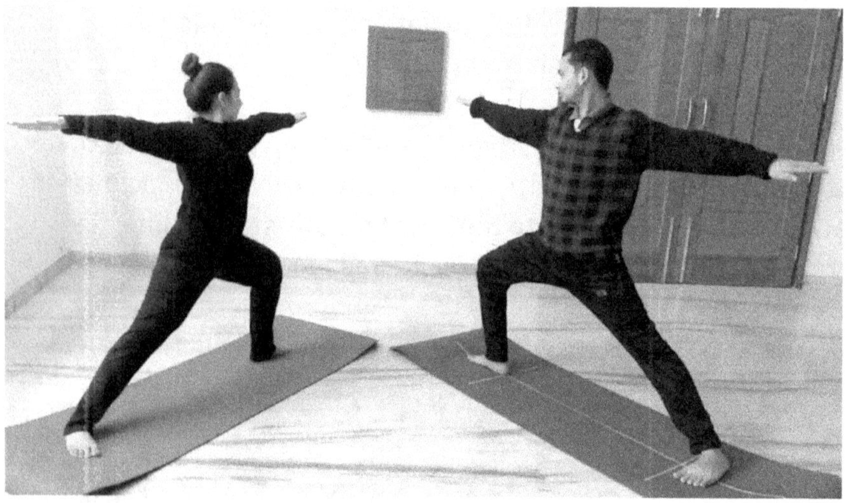

Warrior 2 Virabhadrasana

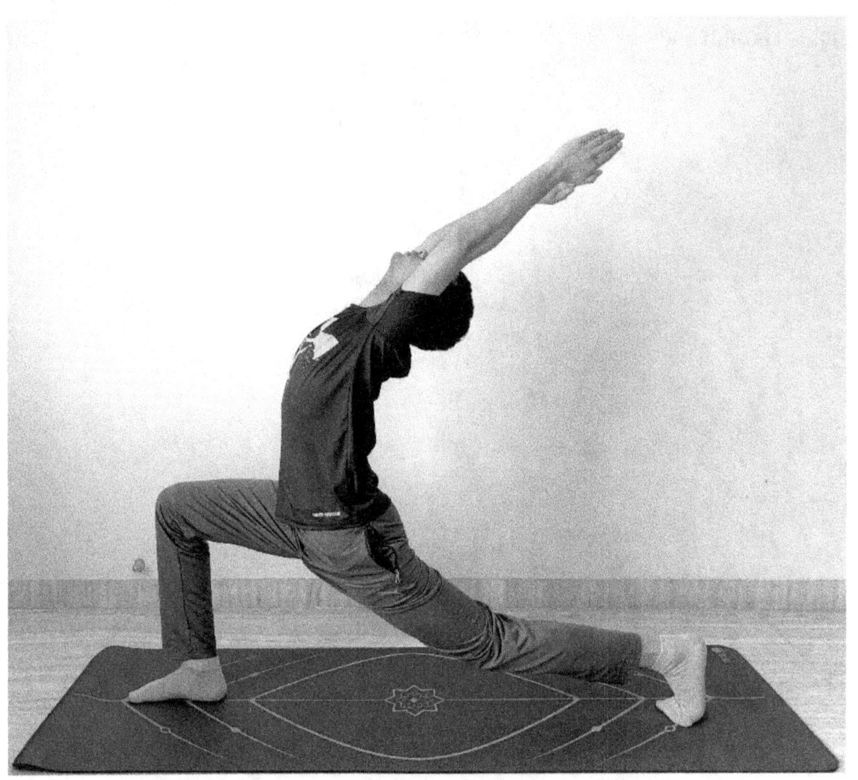

# Triangle Trikonasana

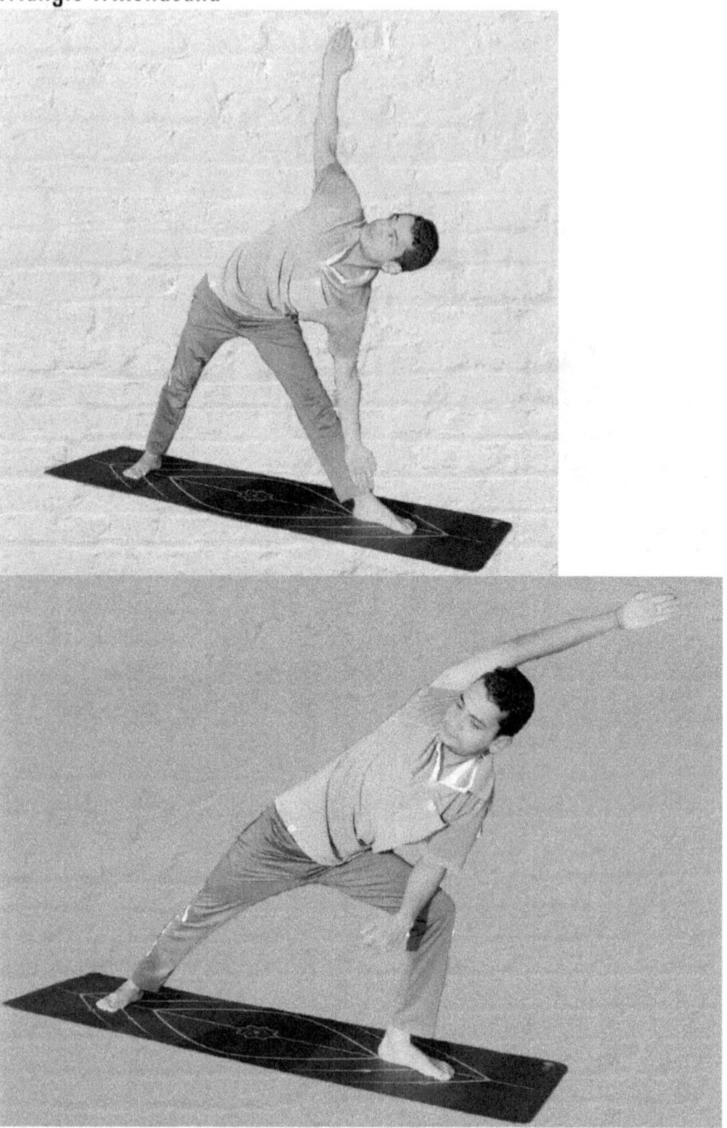

Breathe in and breathe out, hop to bring the feet together.

**Backbend**

Breathe in and breathe out, again position the feet three feet apart and interlock the hands behind the back.

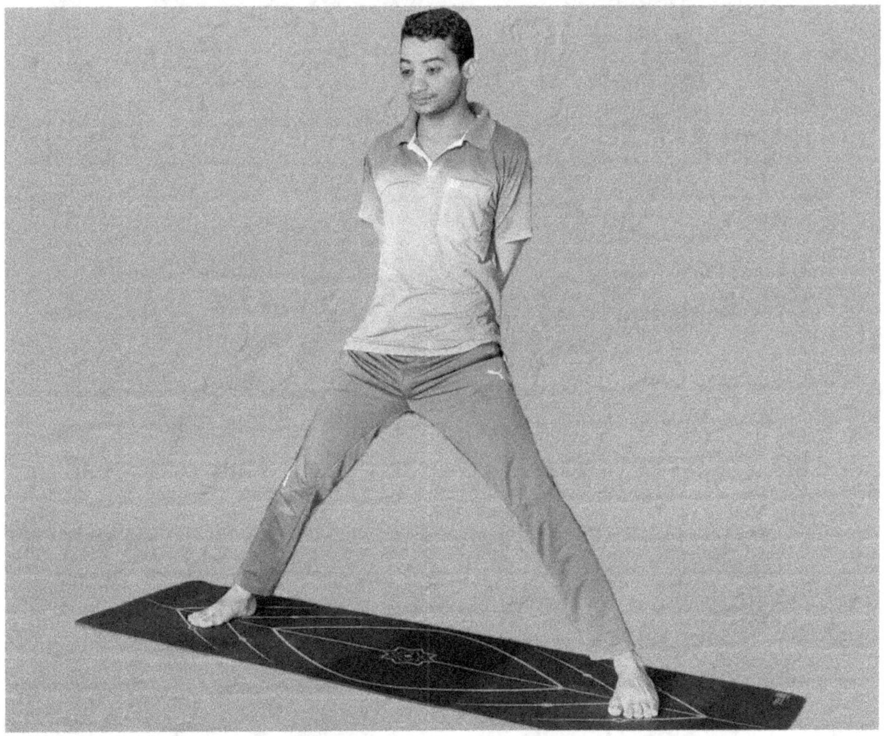

 Inhale and exhale, bend back from the waist.
Push your chest towards the sky.

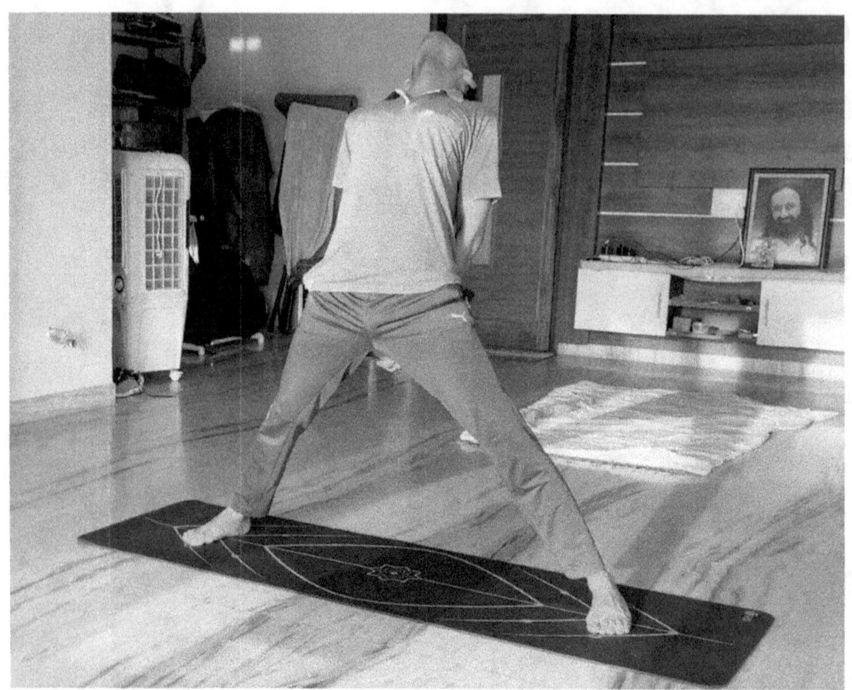

Bend back as far as you can comfortably go, and allow the head to drop further.

Steady the posture for six good breaths.
Inhale center, exhale bend forward from the waist.

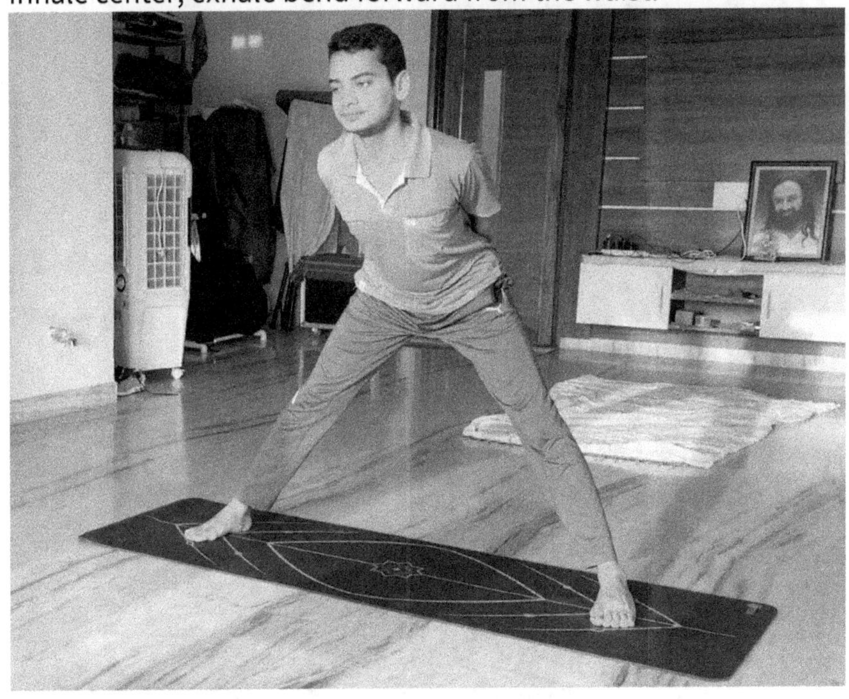

**CLOCK 29 minutes elapsed**
**Forward bend**

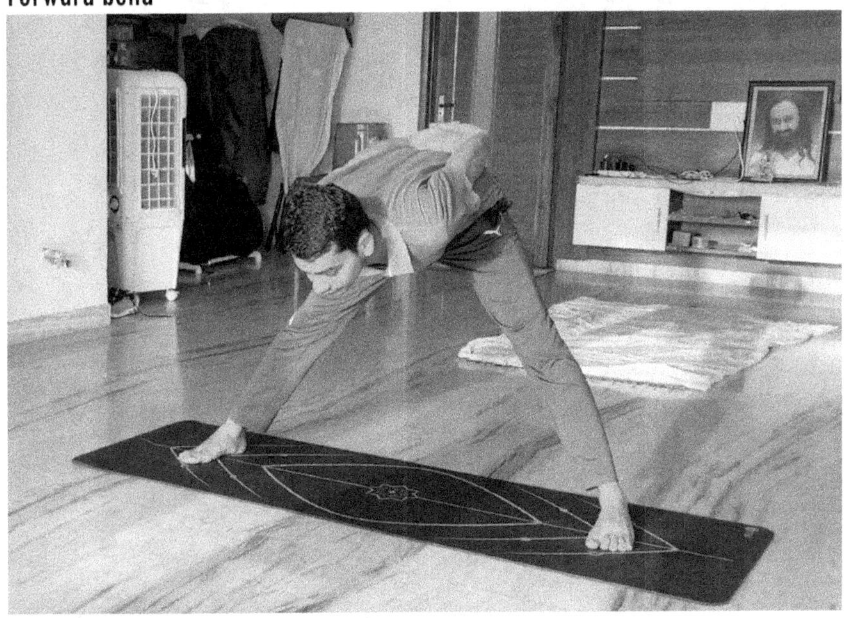

When the waist comes to 90°, start raising the interlocked hands to the top and then hold the posture, stay for six good breaths.

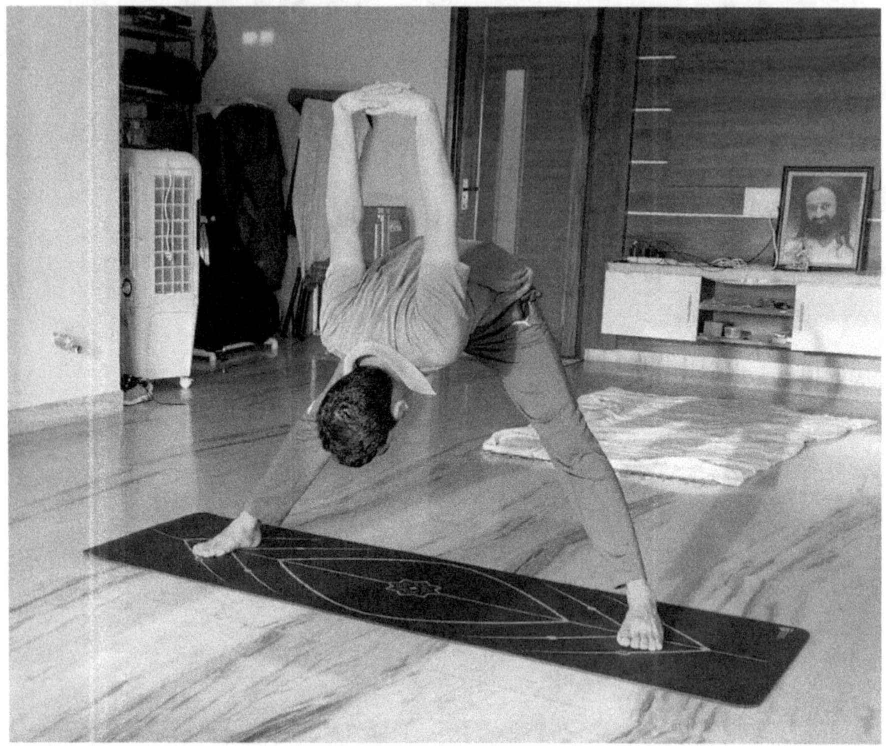

Steady the feet and legs, keep the arms stretched taut, stay in the posture for six good breaths.

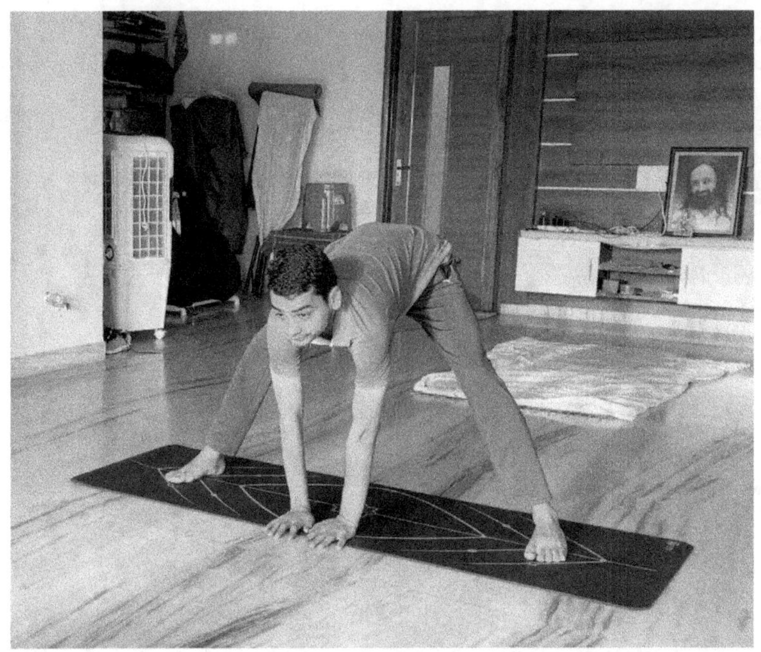

Slowly release the hands, and bring them to rest forward on the floor. Straighten the neck, look front.

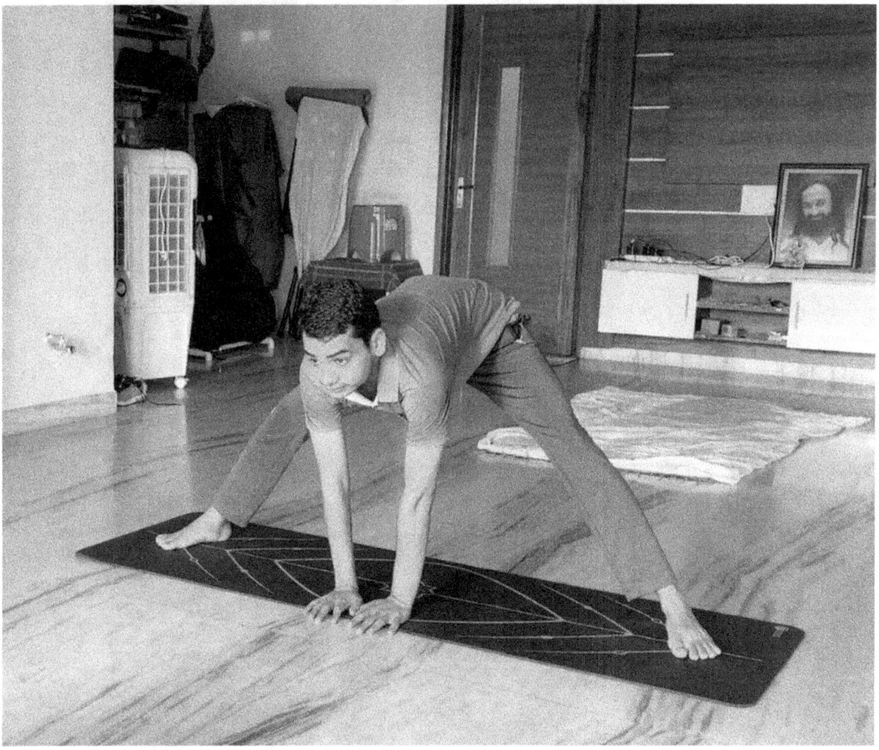

Here, with the support of hands, widen the distance between the feet even more, to maximum. Don't overdo, just extend your comfort zone limits. Stay for six good breaths.

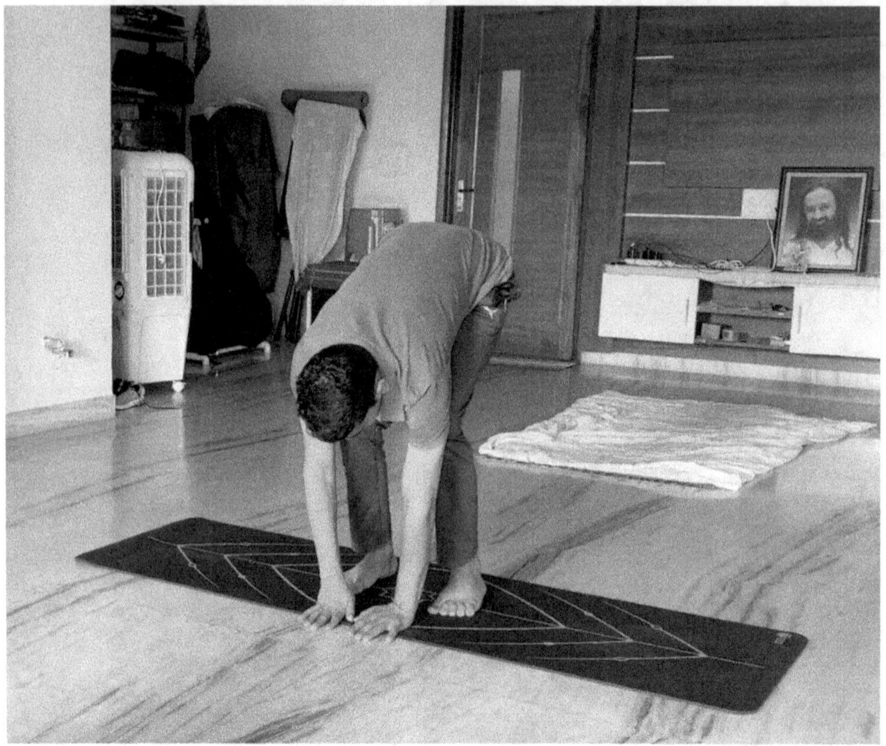

Now slowly walk the feet back to center, keeping the hands in place on the floor. Here the knees may bend some.

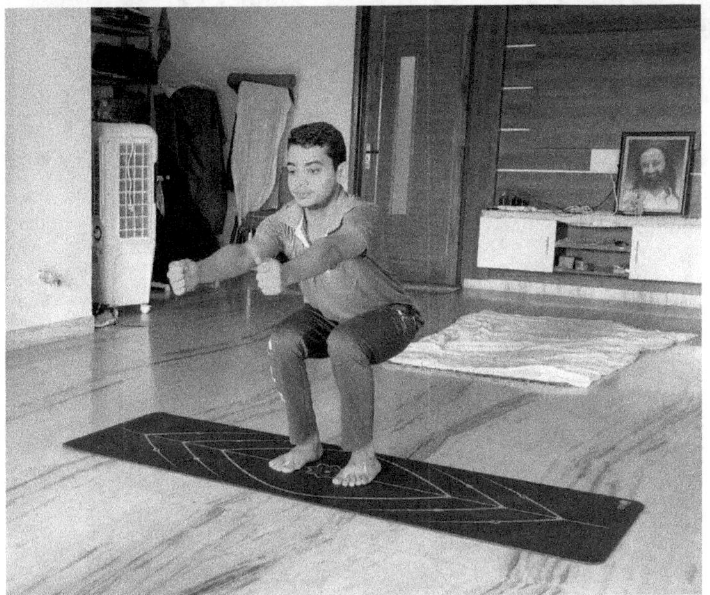

Stretch your arms in front with hands in a fist, and sit on an imaginary chair. Hips back, knees bent, chair pose. Extend the hands in front to steady yourself. Stay for six good breaths.

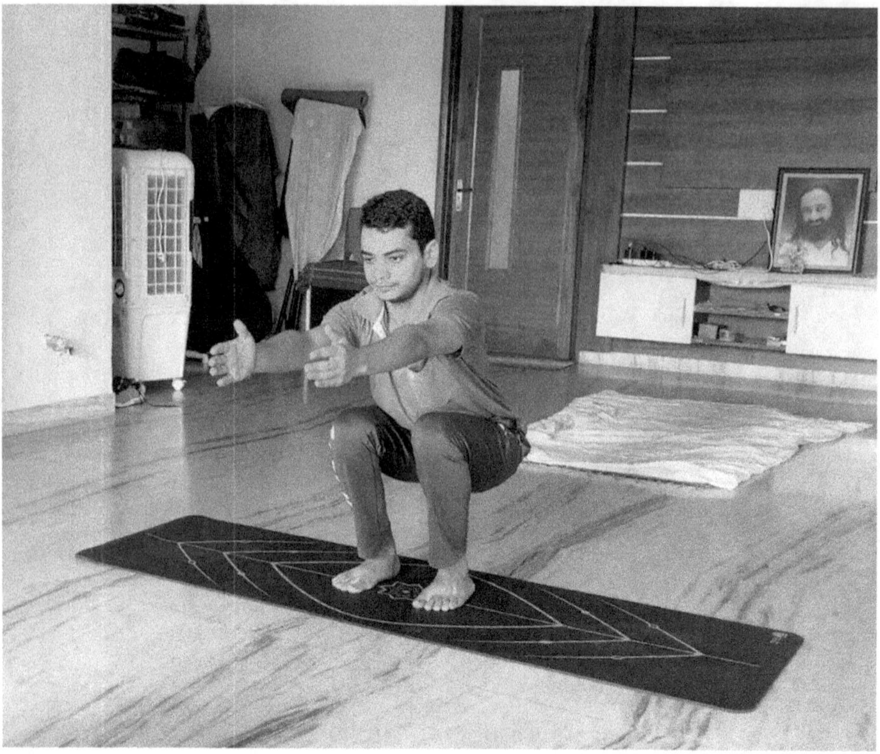

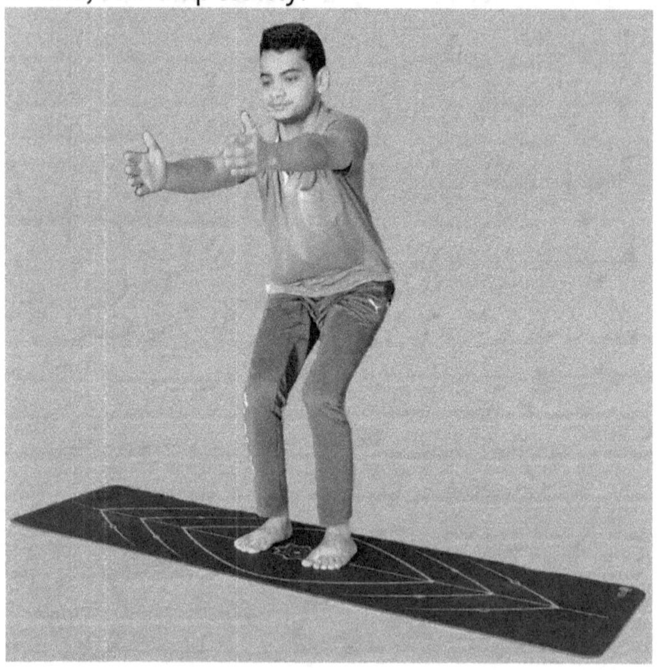

Inhale, stand up slowly.

**Up and Back**

Straighten the spine, take your parallel arms up and back, and
bend back from the waist in a nice arch.

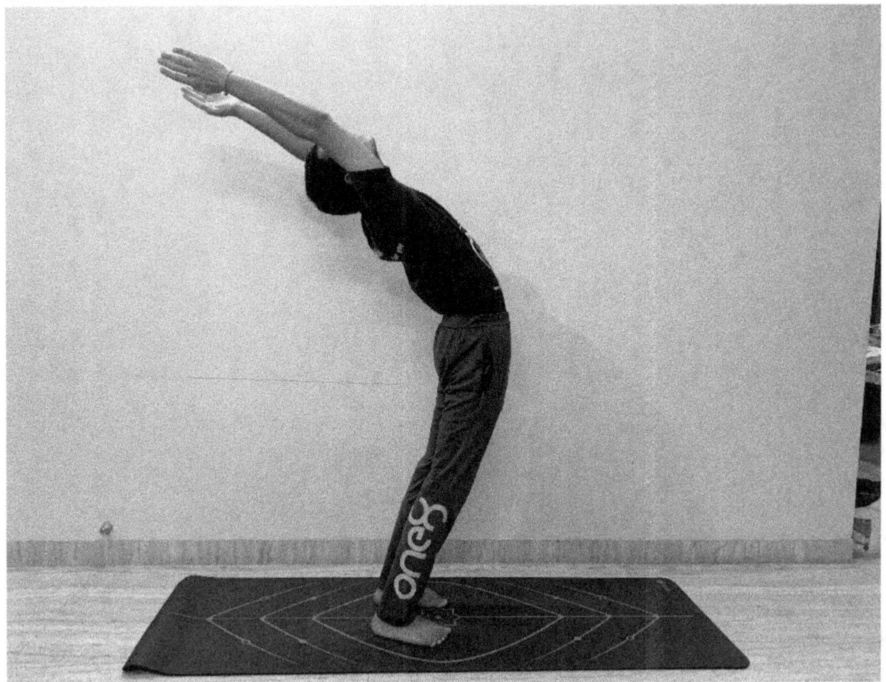

Inhale center, exhale arms come to the sides. Stand straight and
tall.

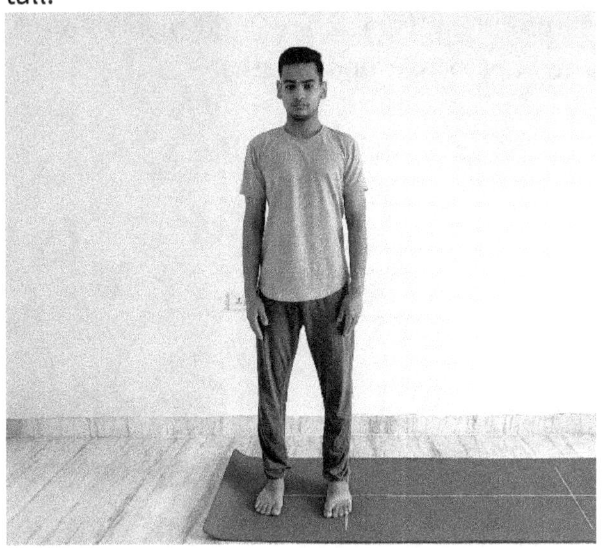

**Sideways Twist**

Again interlock your hands behind the back, twist nicely to the right and stretch the arms taut back at an angle.

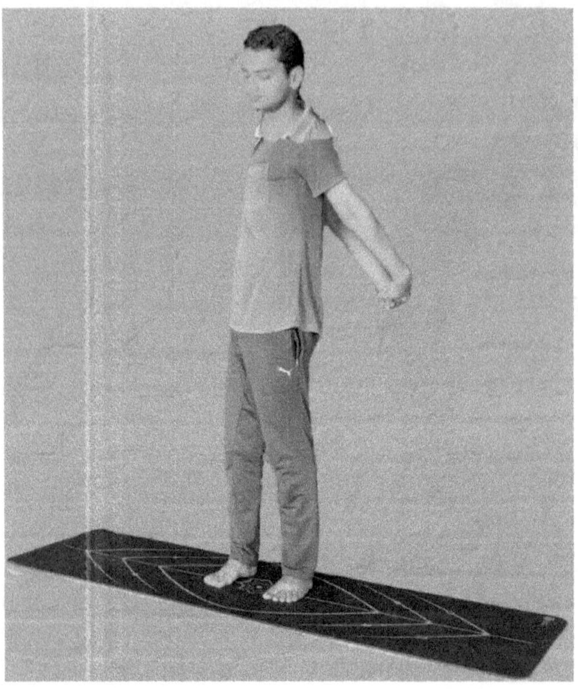

Twist is happening only from the waist, feet are firmly planted on the floor pointing to front. Stay for six good breaths.

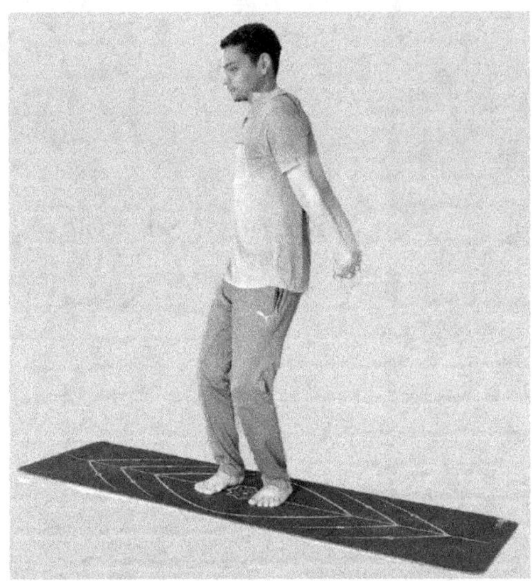

Bend your knees, keep the spine straight, and twist even more.
Then straighten the knees. Stay for six good breaths.

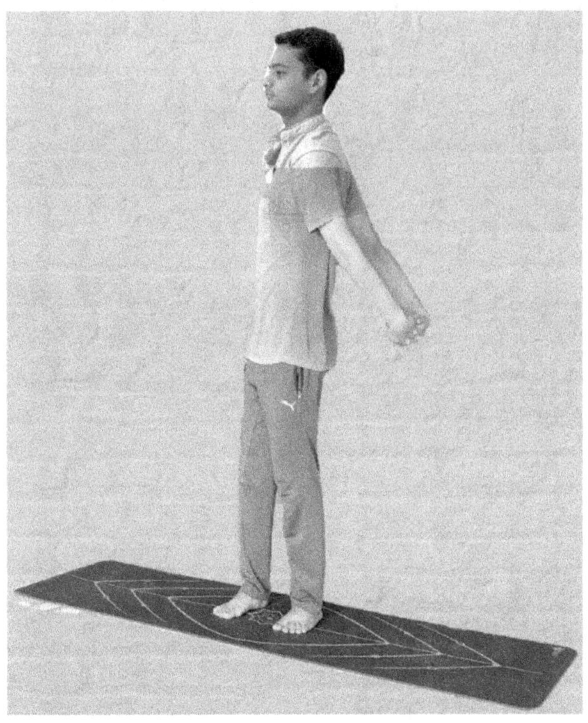

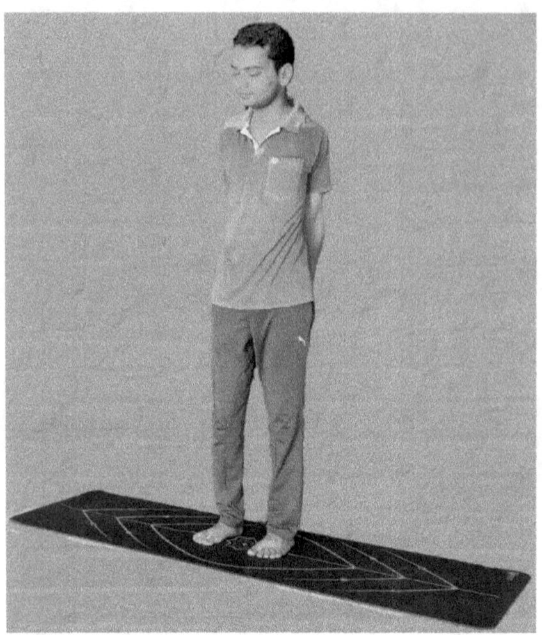

Inhale, come to the center, exhale, twist the other way to the left.

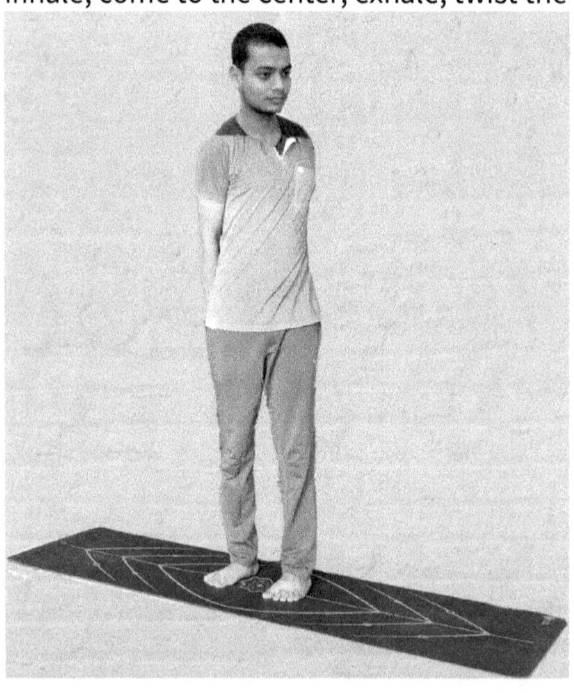

Push your arms back as much as you can, roll your shoulders backwards.

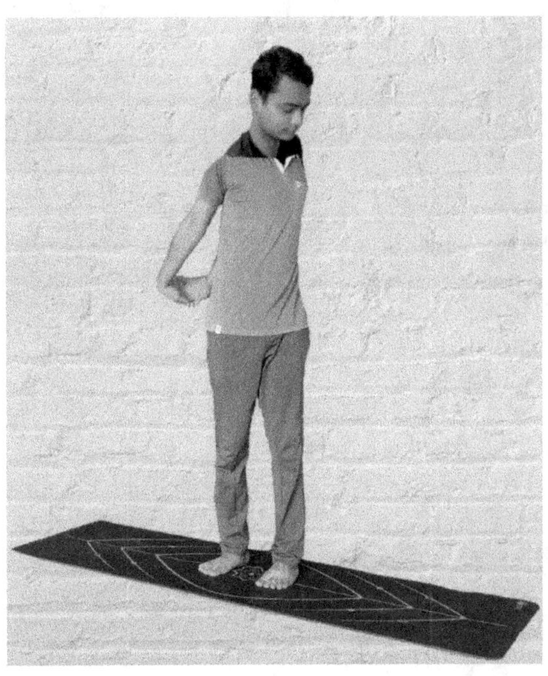

Stay for six good breaths. Then bend the knees and go deeper in the twist, and straighten the knees. Hold the pose for six good breaths.

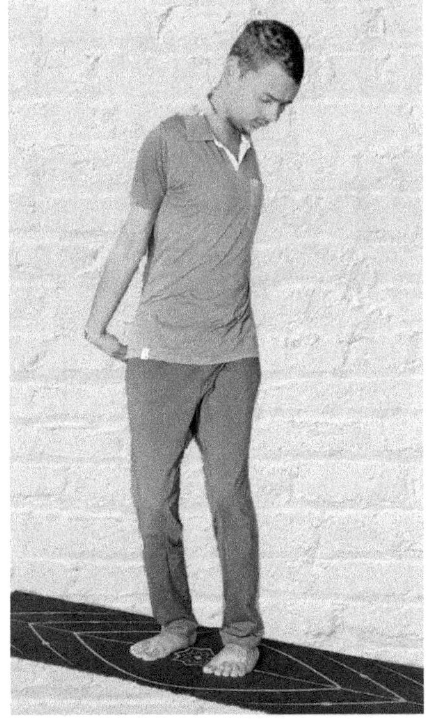

Inhale center, exhale release your arms.


**Shoulder Roll**

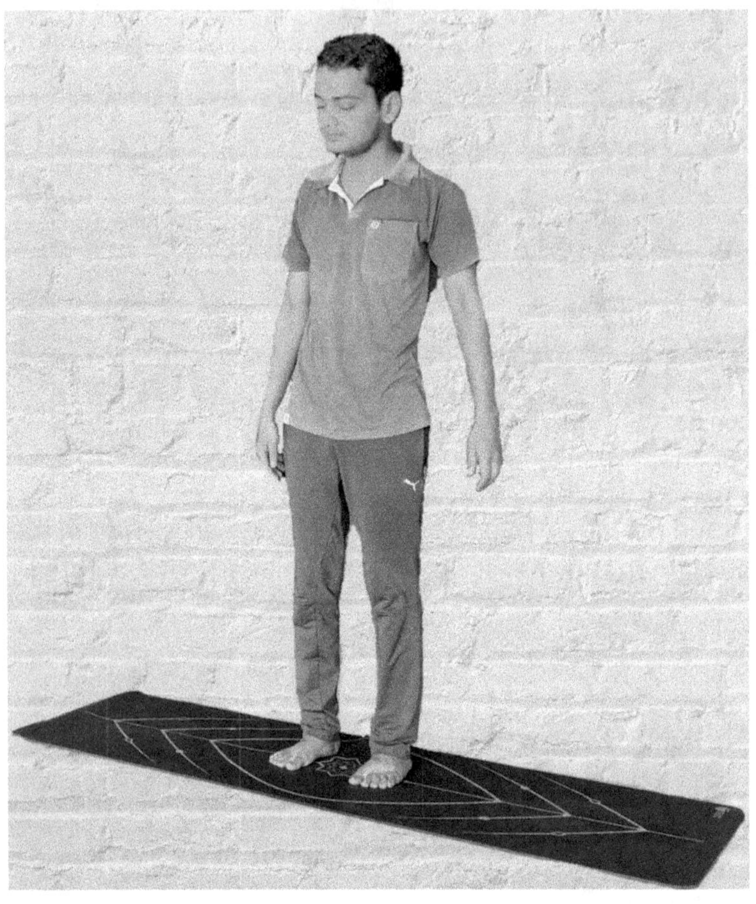

Roll your shoulders clockwise and anticlockwise six times.

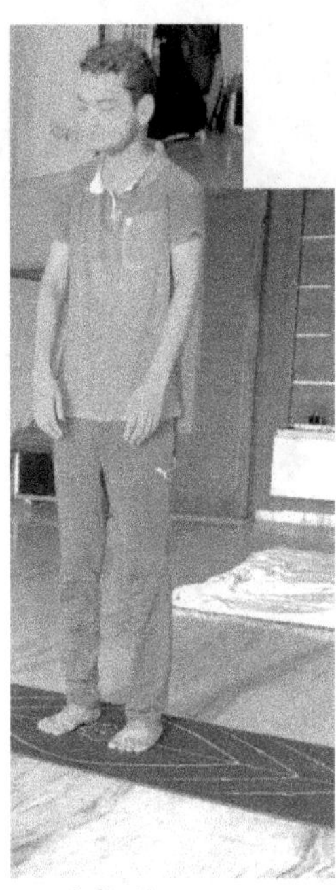

And flail your arms crossing them at the front.

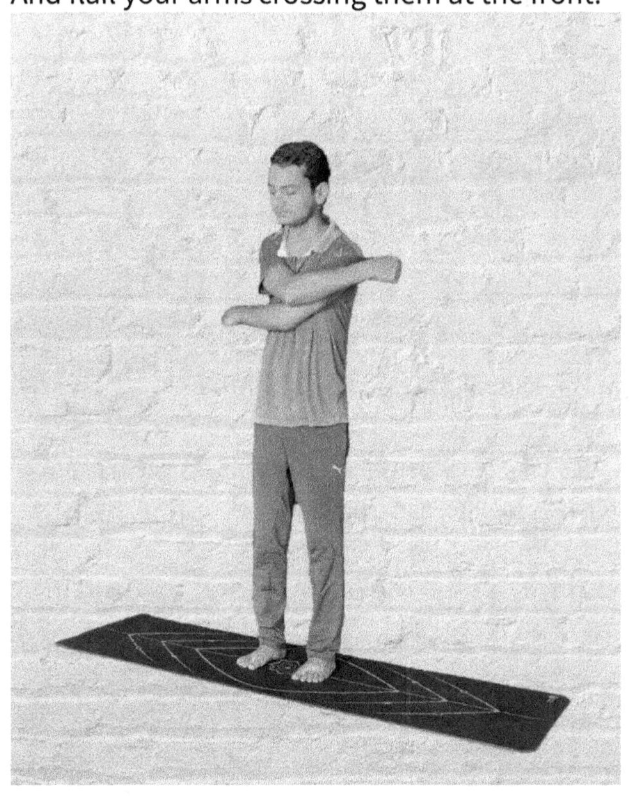

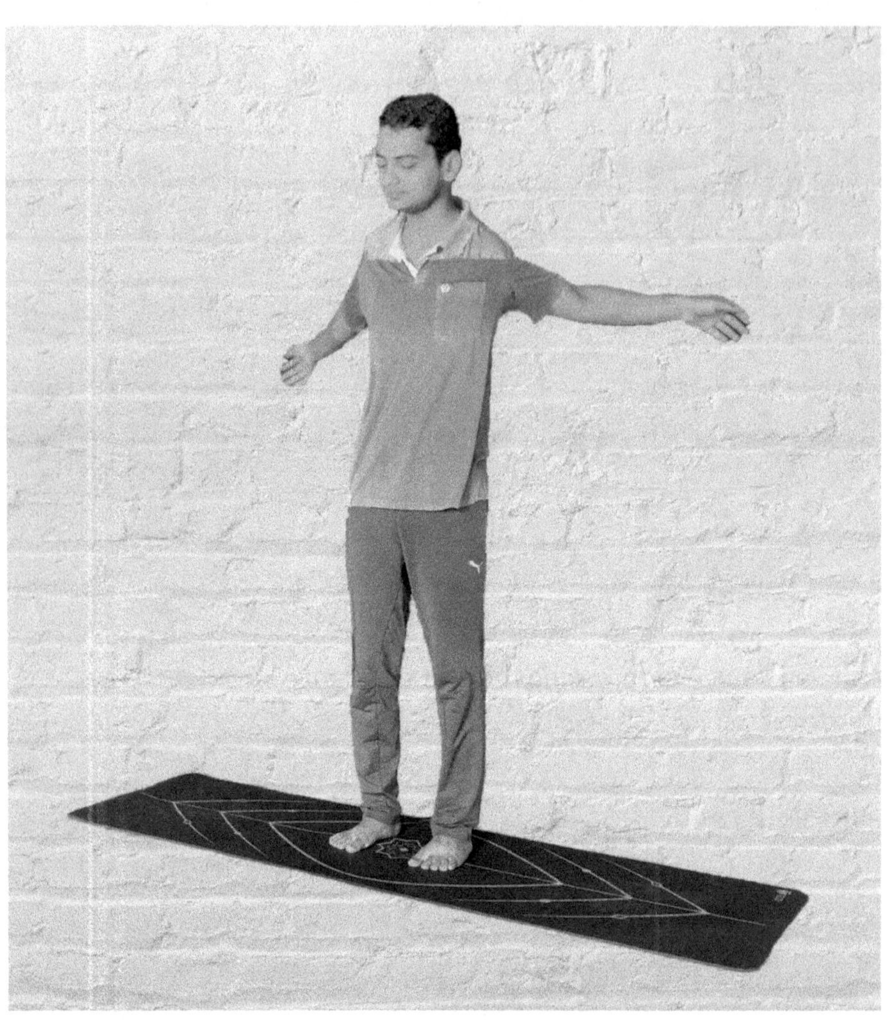

Continue for a minute, then relax. Be still and silent.

Notice your shoulders can take a lot of responsibility, give thanks your knees can support any load, your hands can flex and hold the world.

Gently we may sit down in Malasana the potty squat.

**Malasana the lightness, cheerfulness, ready for anything stance**

Sit on your haunches a foot apart, interlock your hands, arms stretched to front.

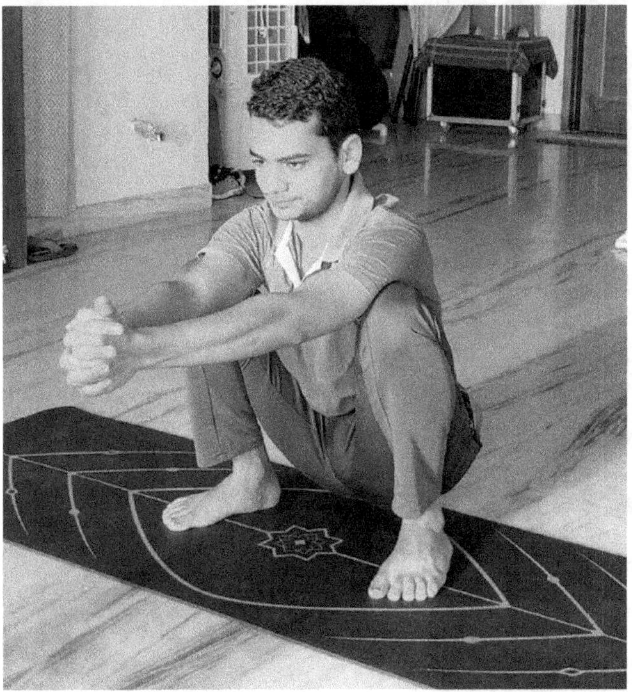

Inhale, take your arms up, and raise your head and look up at your hands.

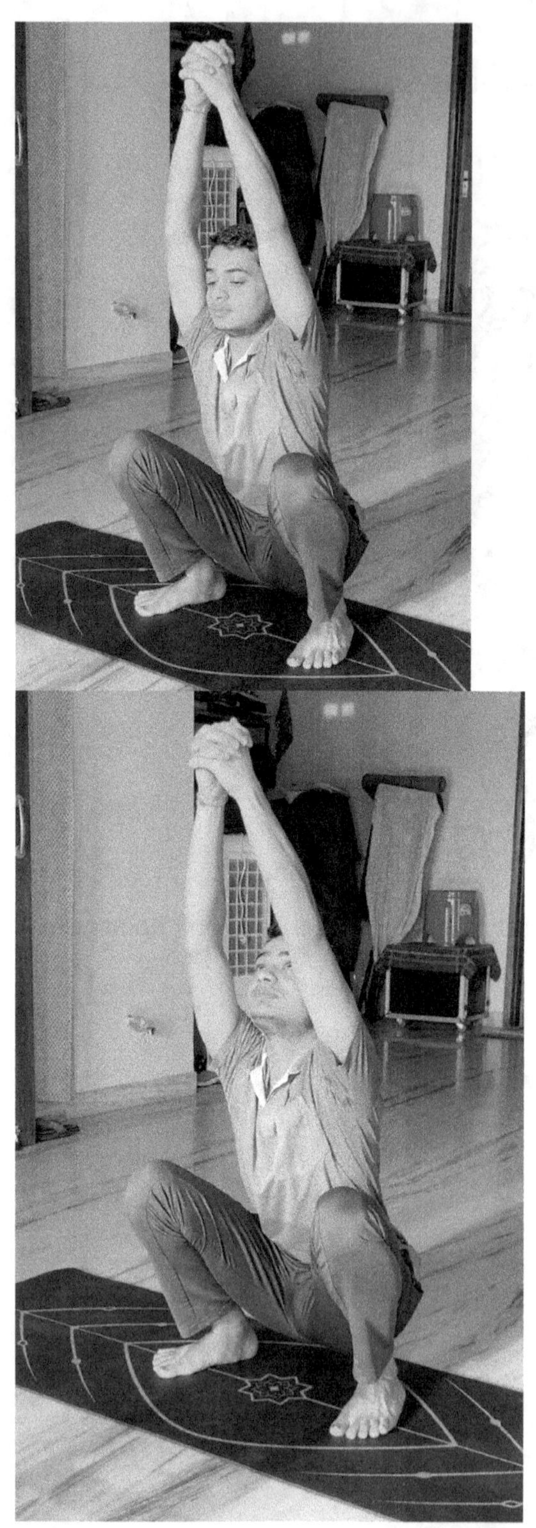

Exhale and bring the arms forward and down while loudly saying "Ha" sound.

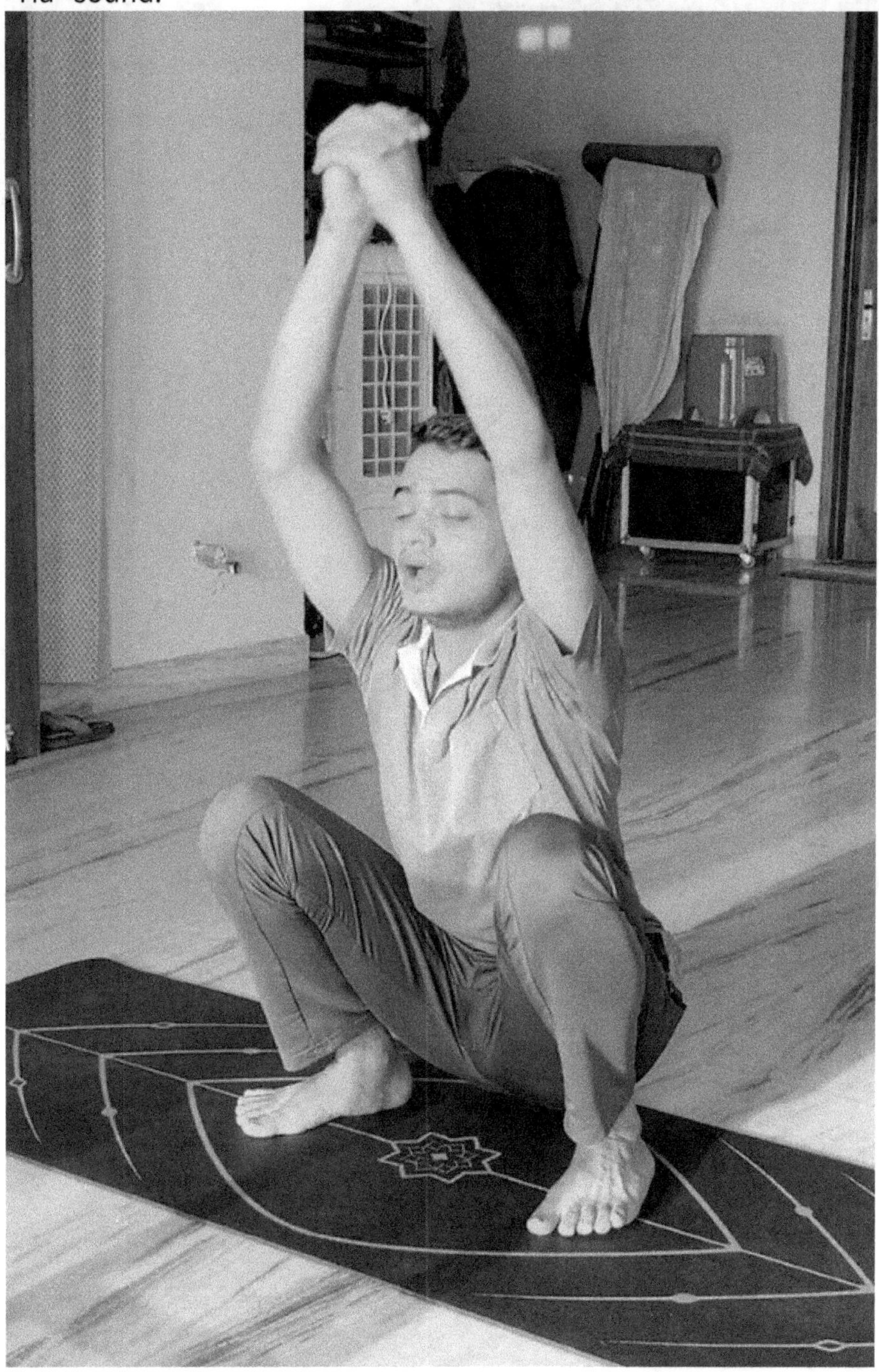

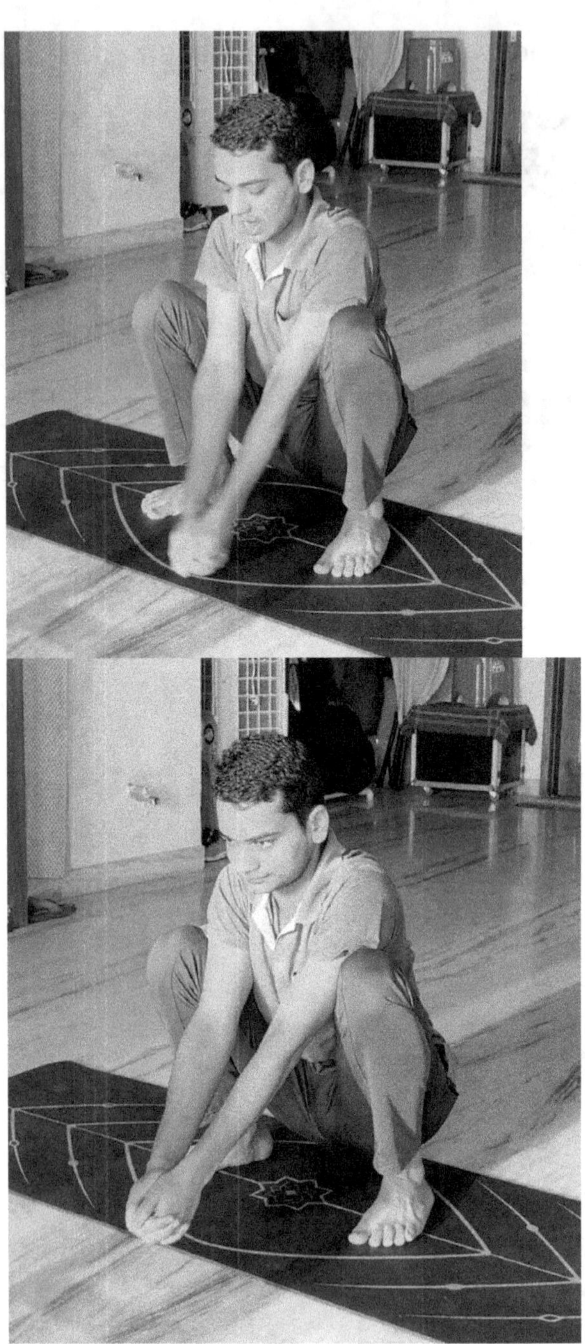

Continue the "Ha" sound and arm movements six times, with deep lungful each time.

Release the posture, and gently come into Vajrasana.

CLOCK 39 minutes elapsed
Namaste behind the back for enhanced acceptance, ok in the face of defeat and
ready to drop smile and move on

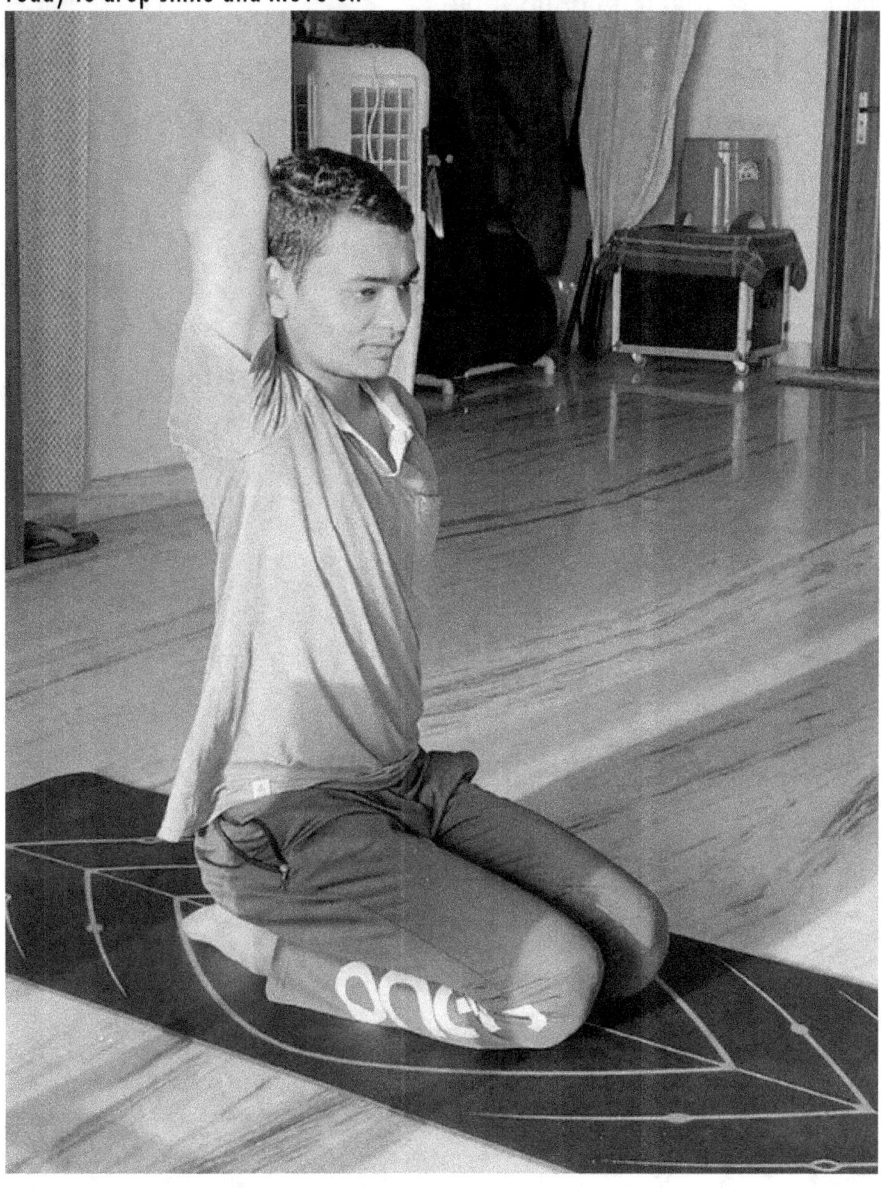

Sitting in Vajrasana, take the right arm up and back, take the left arm to clasp the right hand behind the back. Maintain the steady posture for six good breaths.

Release and repeat the other side, with the left arm on top. Adjust your neck so that it is comfortable.

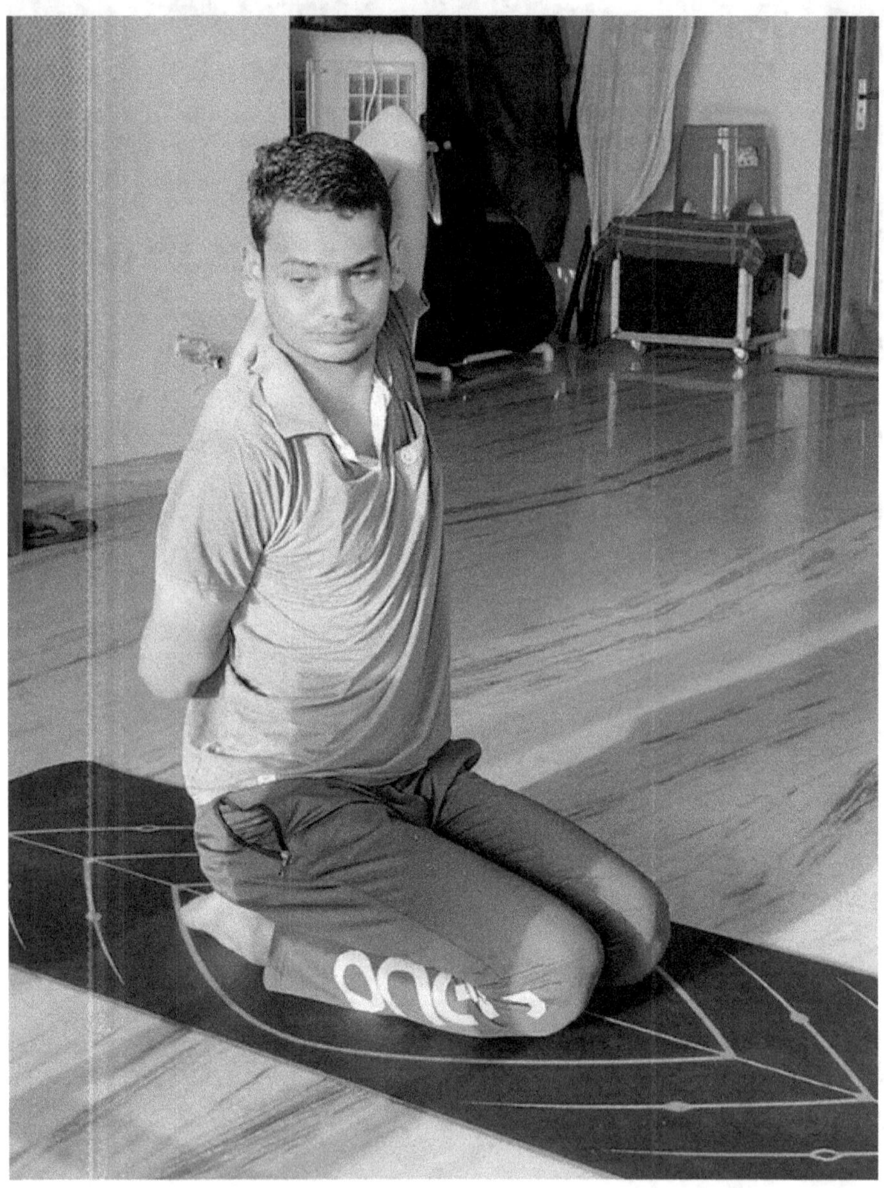

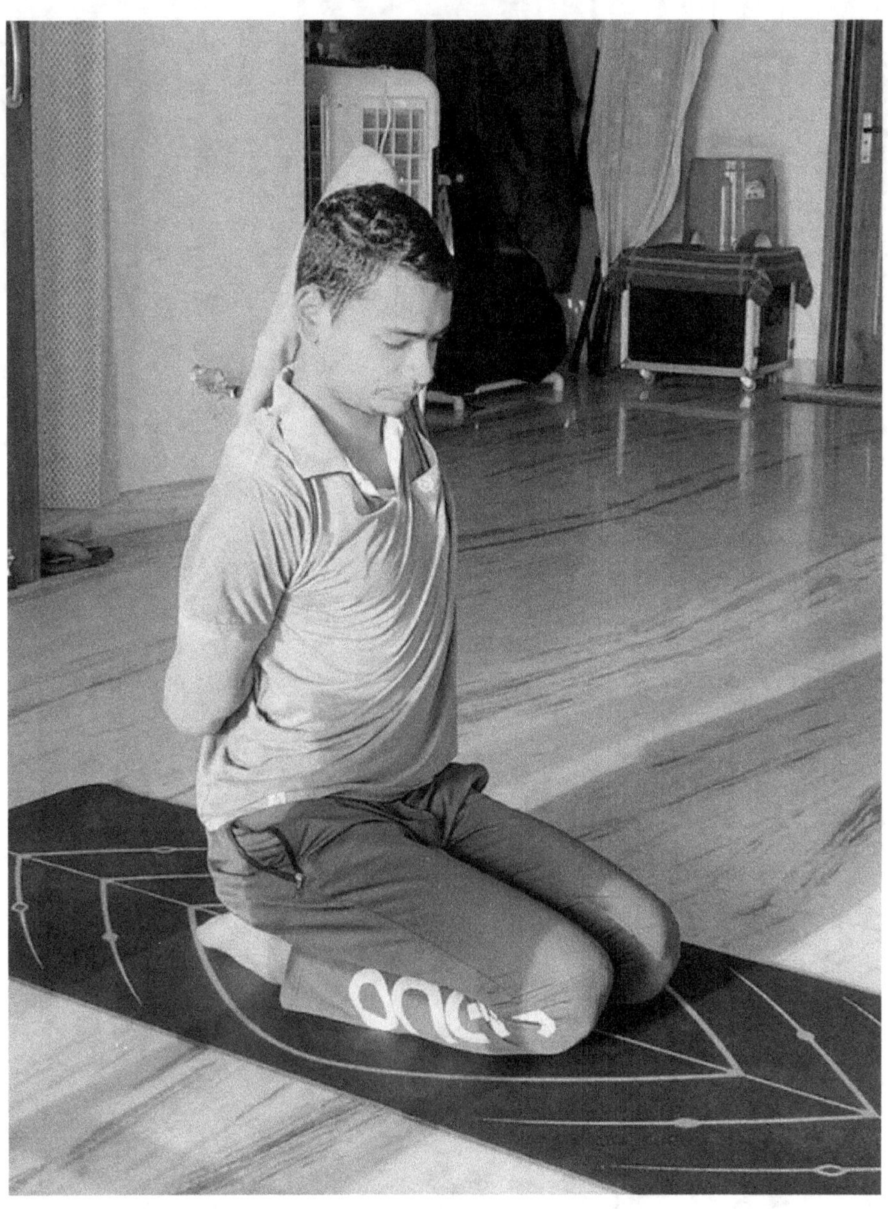

Release. Come forward, elbows on the floor, cross your arms, hold your biceps.

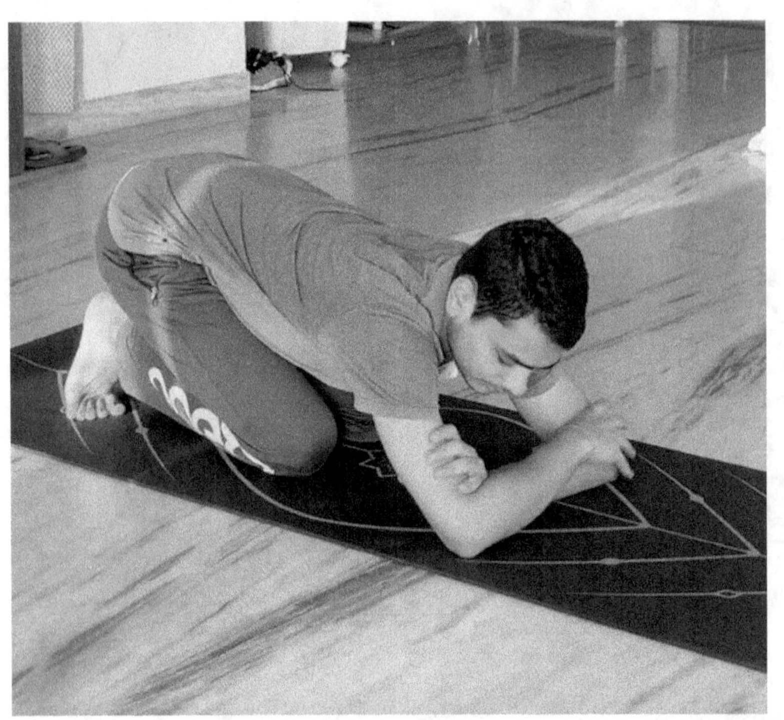

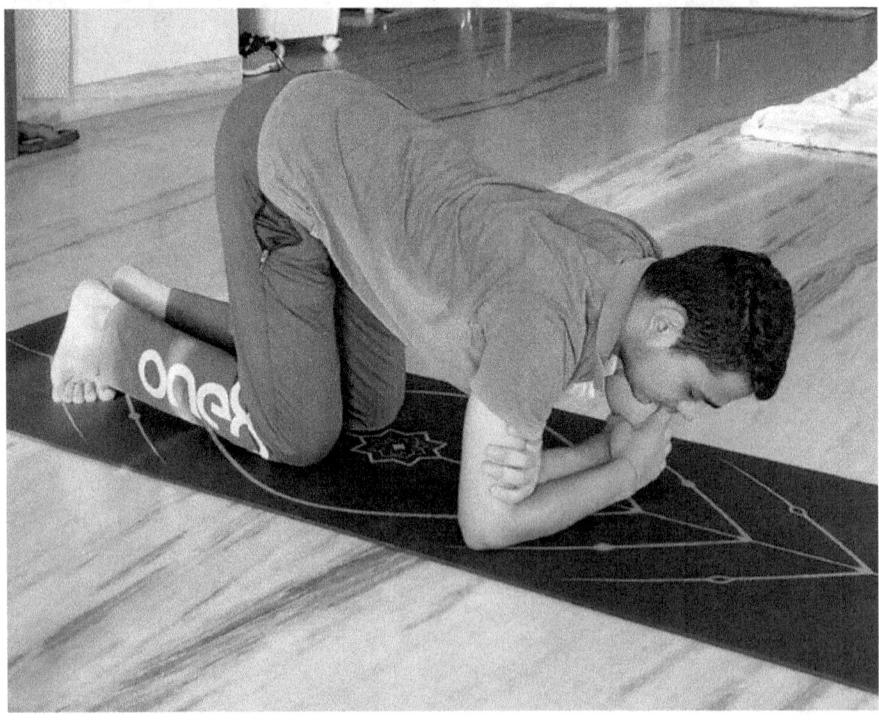

Inch forward, take your legs back, lie down on top of your arms.

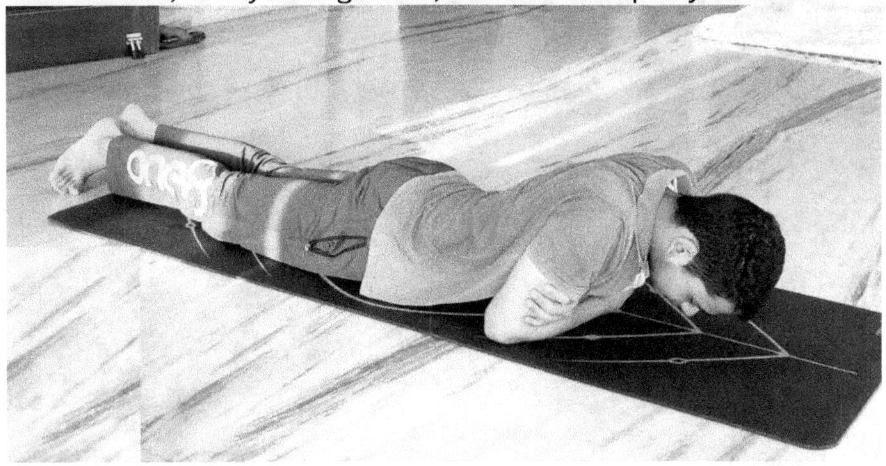

Take your forehead down, your hips are down.

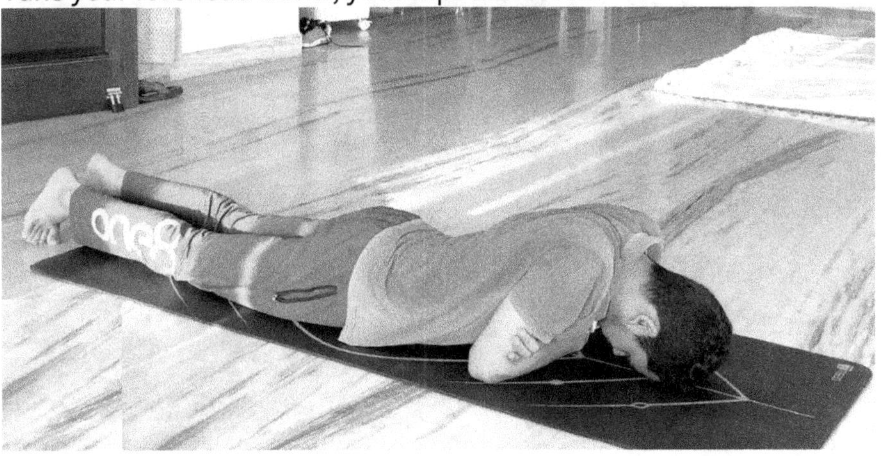

Inhale and come up. Lift your chest up, hips up, feet firmly planted, elbows on the ground. May move the neck a bit to make it comfortable.

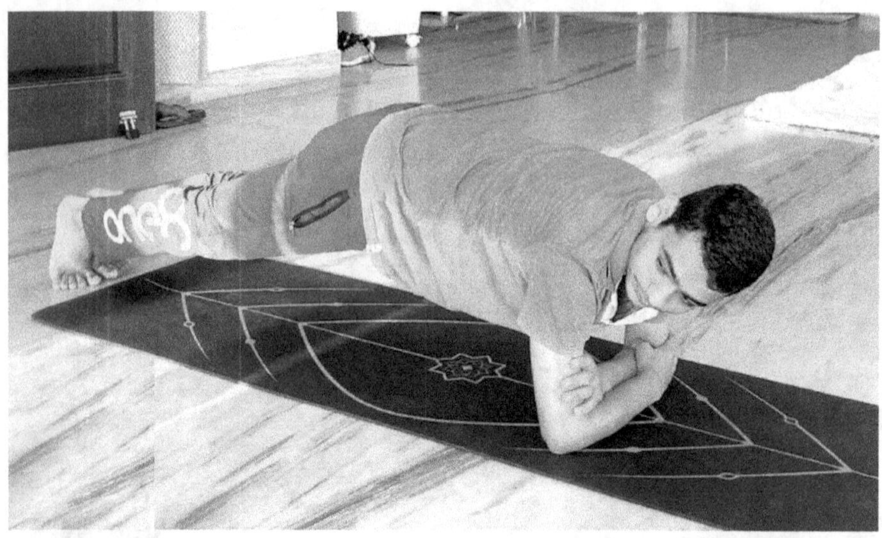

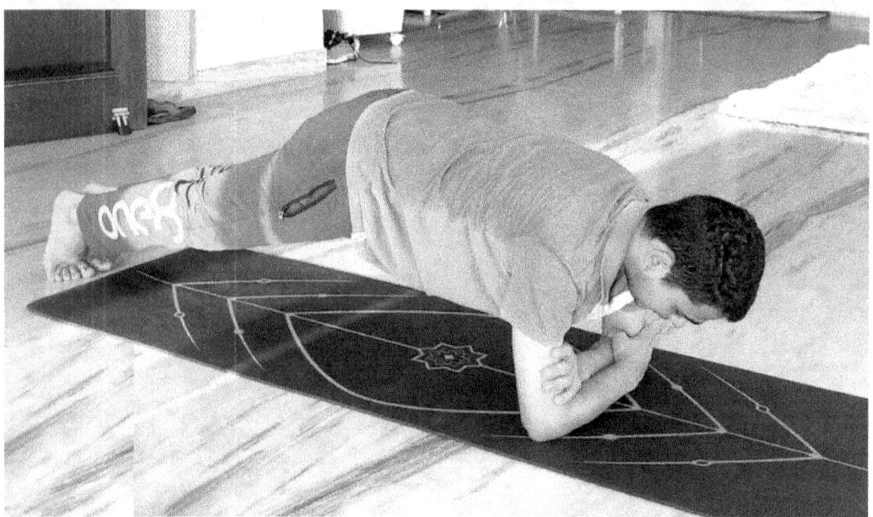

Inhale, knees come down to the floor, hips raised, slide back to place your chin on the floor just near the arms, nose almost touching.

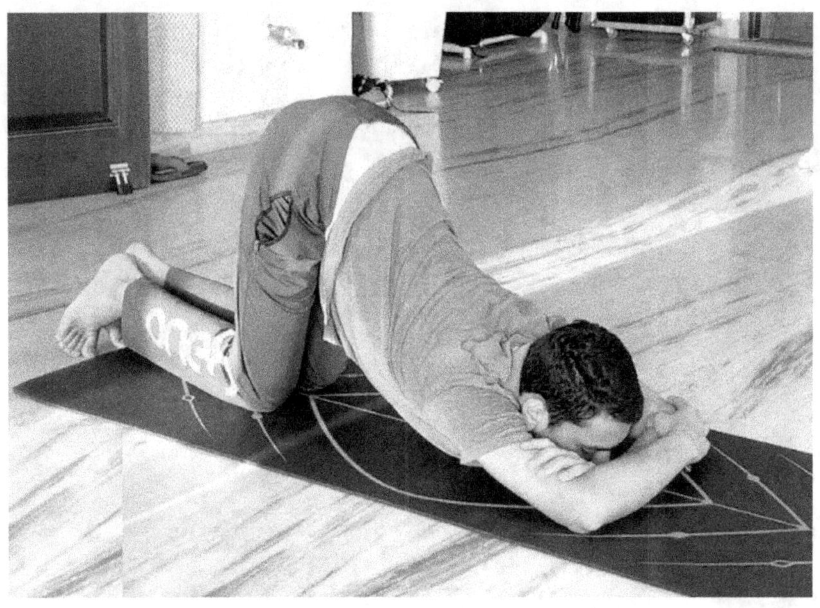

Ready to accept and forgive, forget... are the dynamic principles that keep you safe and whole

Inhale and come up, as if bracing for the event.

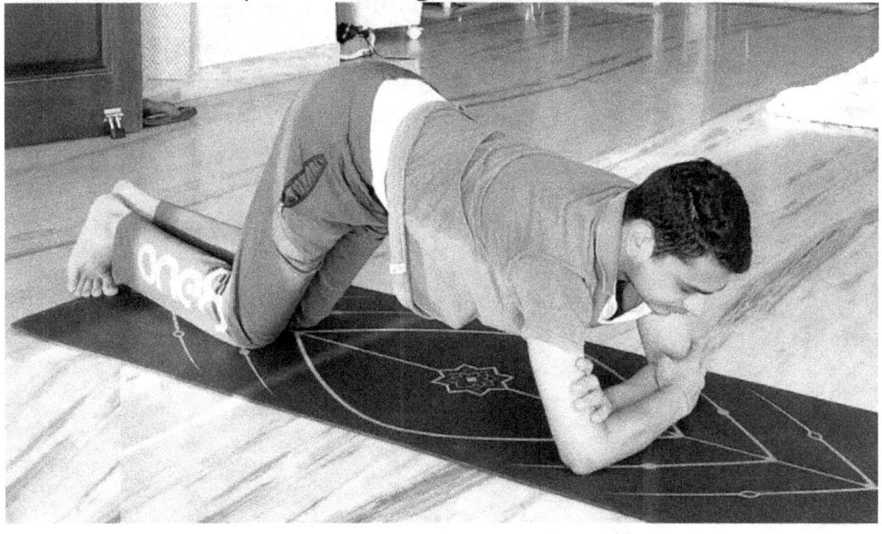

Go forward and down all the way, hips down, head down, feet together.

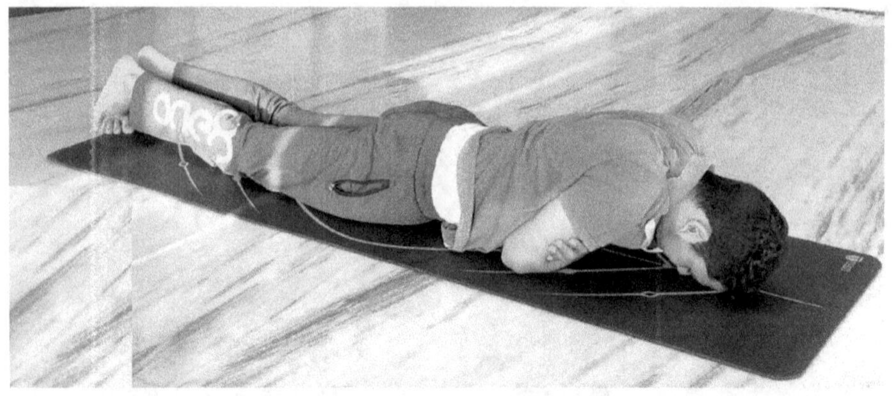

Inhale come up to plank pose.

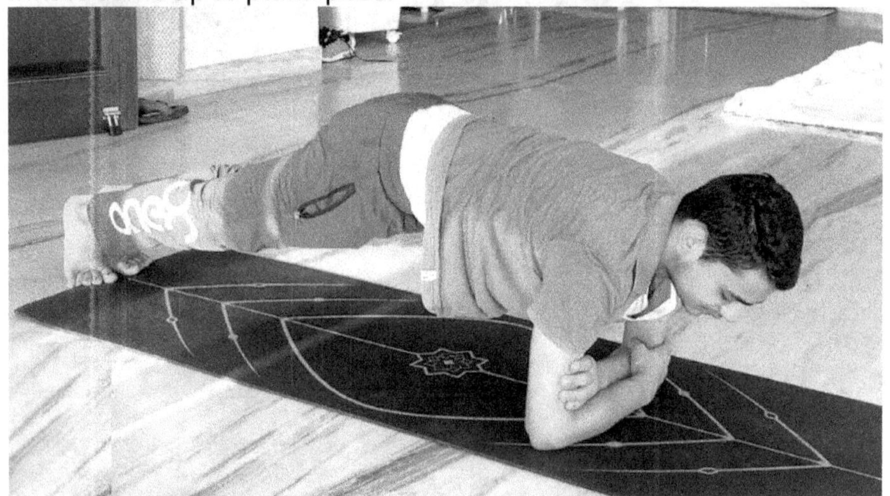

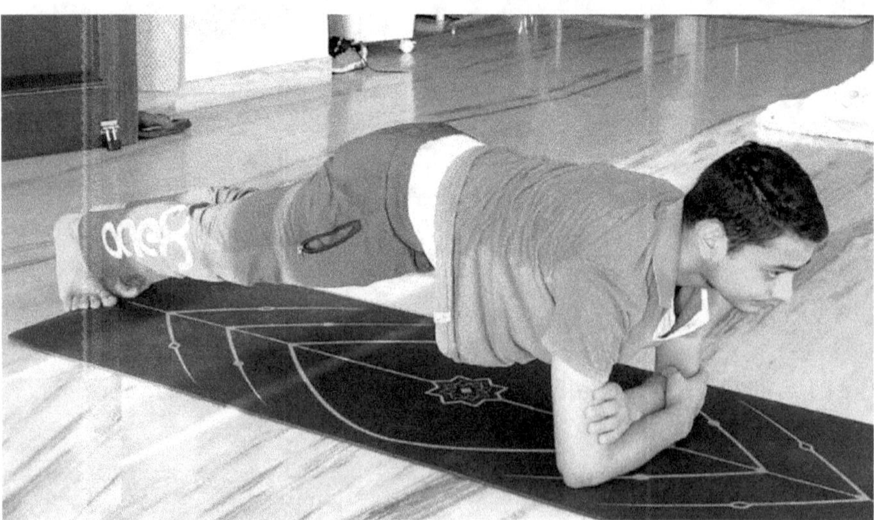

Plank means you are supple and strong and well off to maintain a family and keep your house together.

Inhale and exhale, and bring the knees to the ground, and chin to the floor behind the arms.

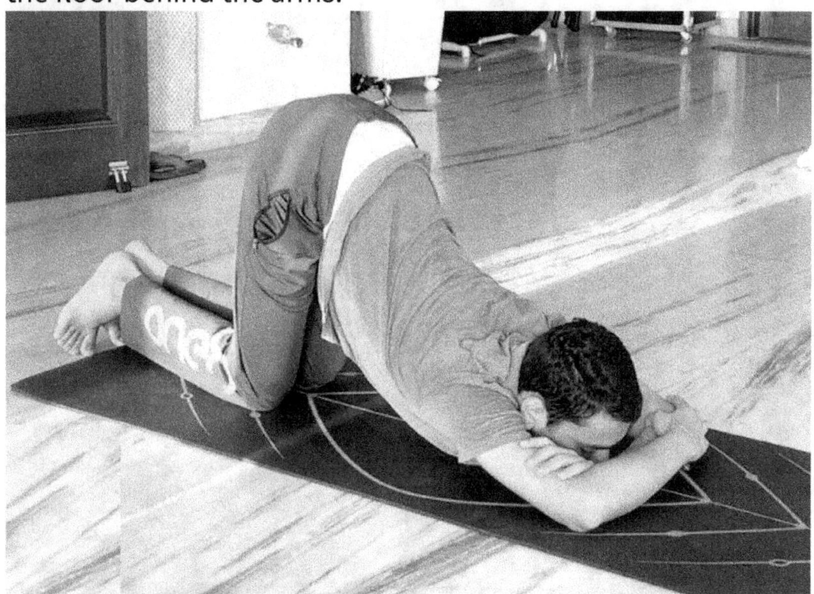

If you are unwilling to lose, you can never win...OPPOSITE VALUES ARE COMPLEMENTARY IN NATURE

CLOCK 43 minutes elapsed
Bow
Inhale and release, unlock your arms. SPHINX Pose (or we may do the traditional bhujangasana cobra pose).

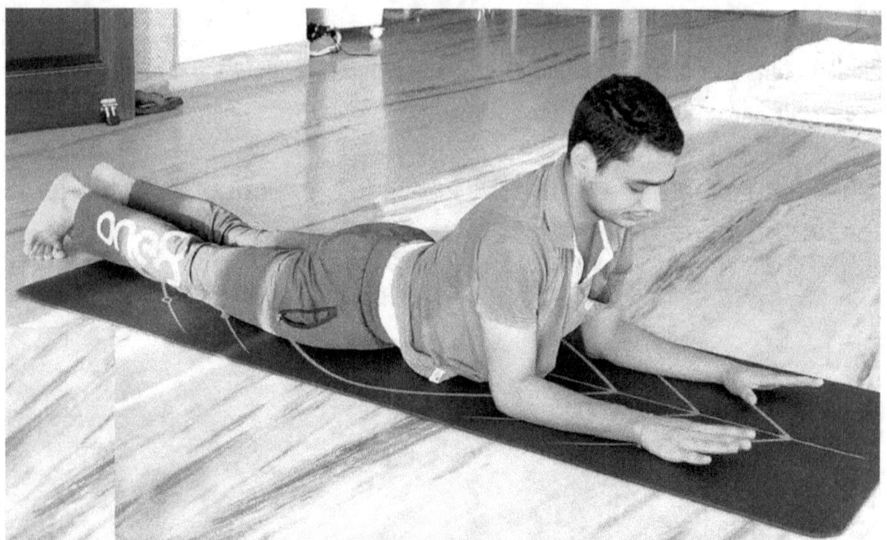

Elbows are aligned to your shoulders, bent at 90°. Forearms on the floor, feet together.

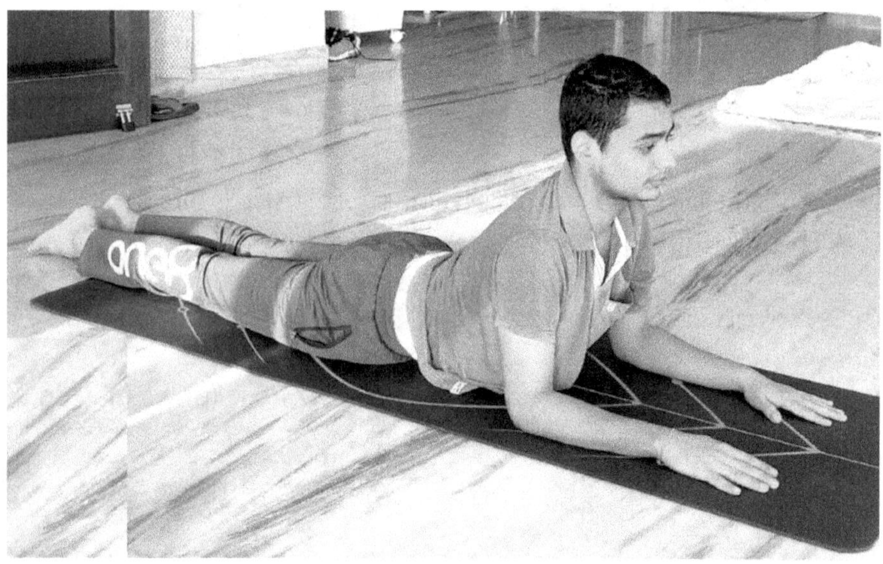

Inhale, lift your head up, look up. Imagine you are pushing your chest out from in between the shoulders. As if someone is pushing your spine from behind.

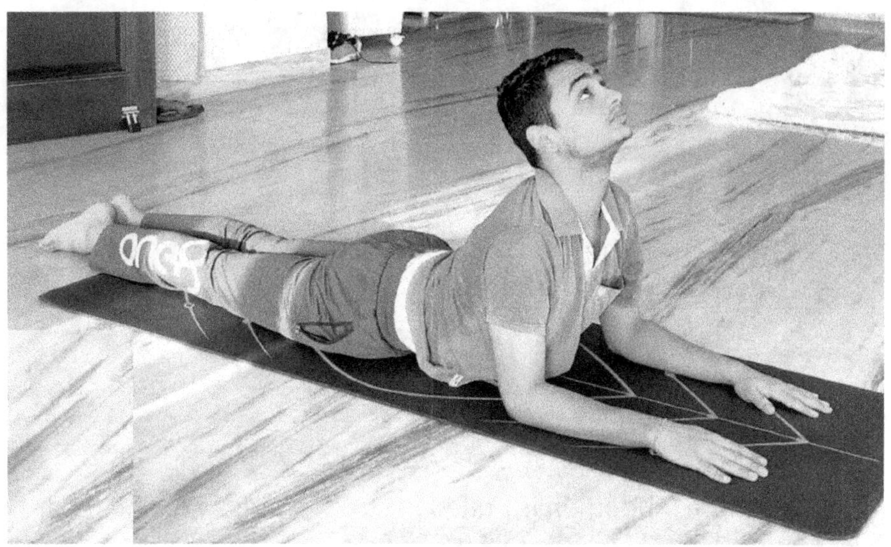

Take your head back just a little bit more. Keep your arms strong, don't shrug your shoulders.

Engage the abdomen muscles, pull the navel in. engage your pelvic floor, contract, and take your head back even more for a nice arch in the spine. Hold steady for six good breaths.

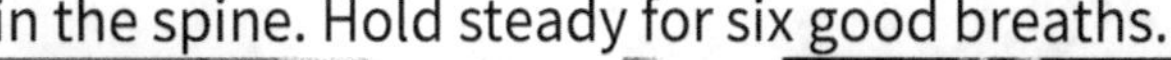

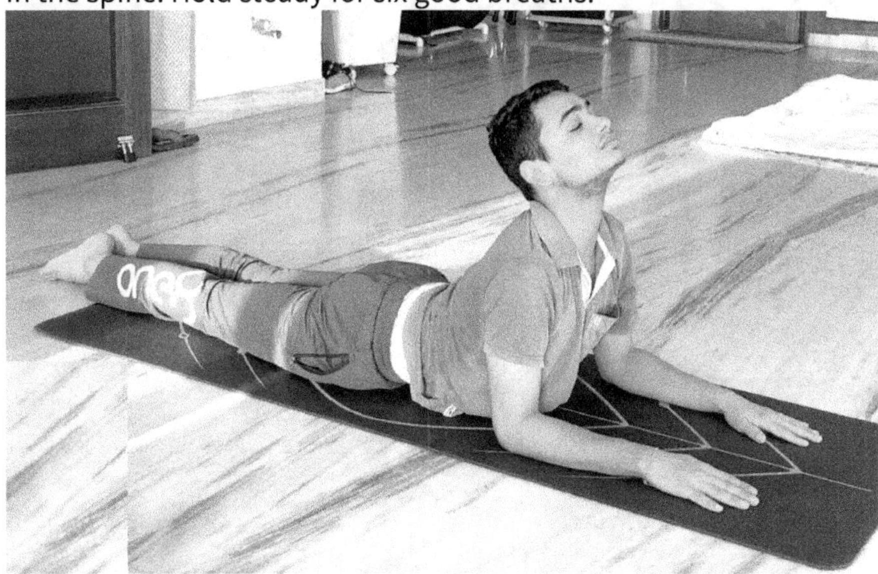

Slowly straighten your elbows.

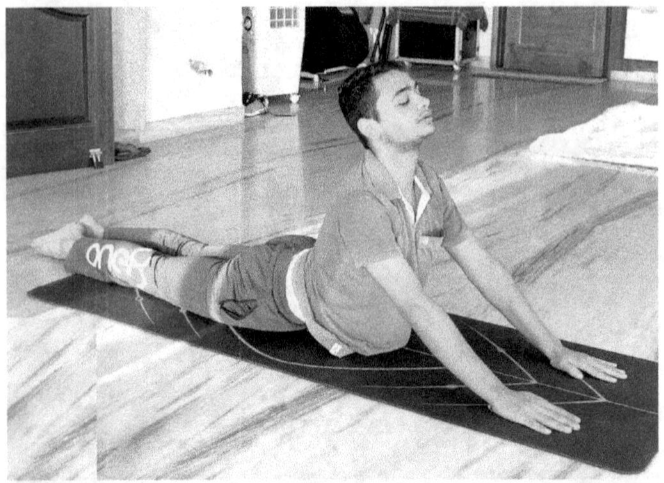

Arch even more. Abdomen is pulled in strongly. Legs are engaged.

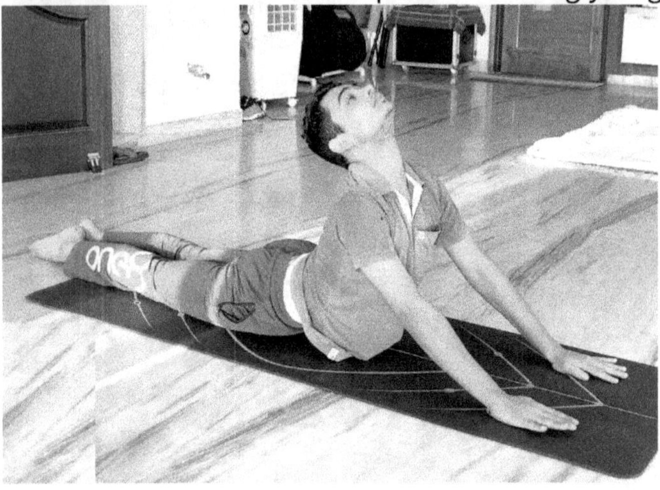

As you exhale, first the elbows come down to the floor.

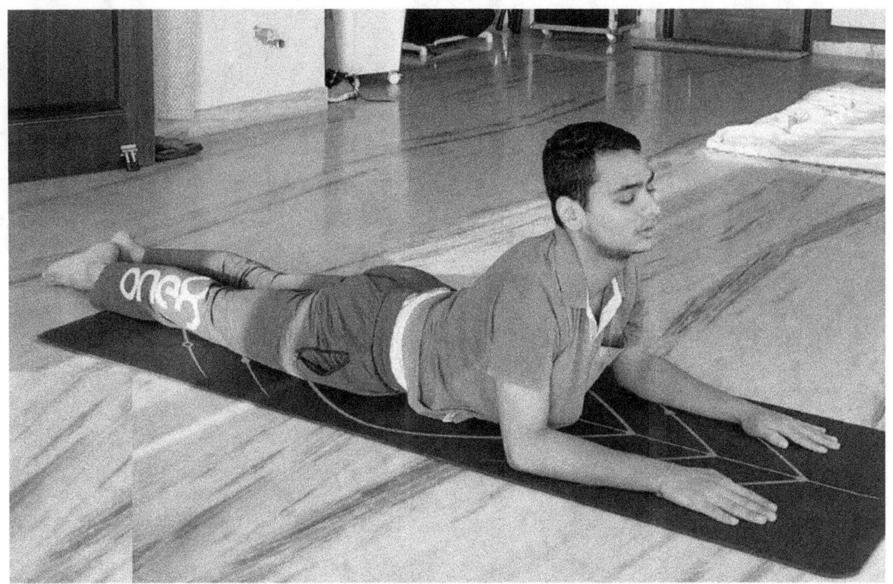

Then very slowly, adjust your arms and head goes down one side on the floor.

CLOCK 44 minutes elapsed
**Makarasana**

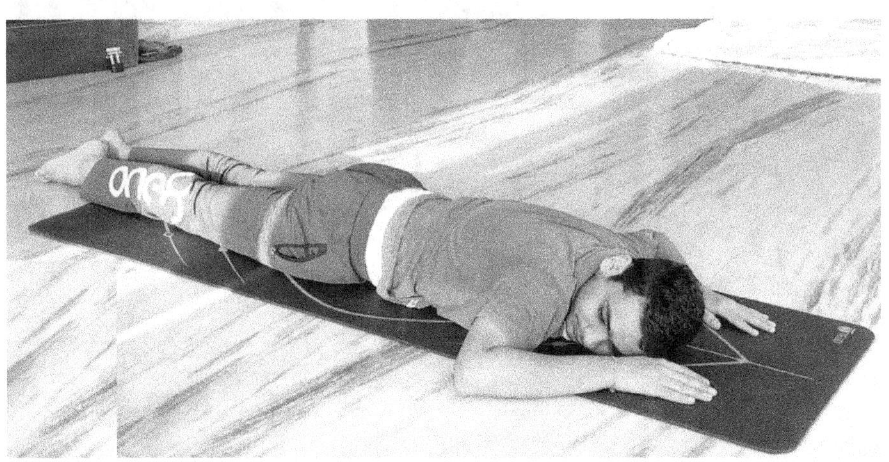

**Bow**

Move your hands back to grab the ankles. First you lift your head
up, chest up. Adjust your ankle hold better. Knees comfortable.
Inhale bring your legs off the ground. Balance yourself on the nabhi.

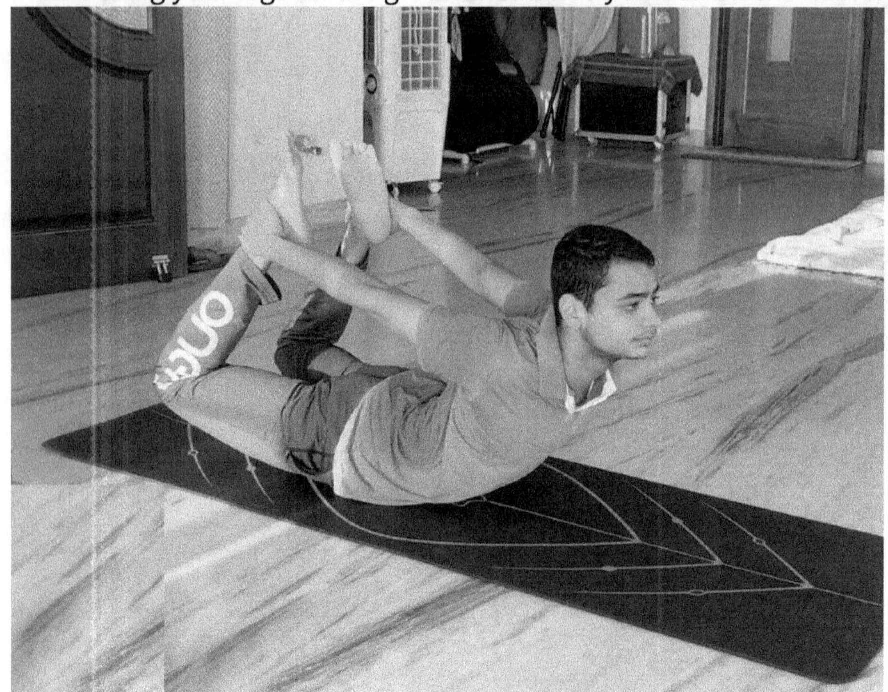

**Supta Vishnu**

Close your eyes, let your body be limp. Adjust yourself and become more comfortable. Keep your neck in the center or to a side. Release any strain from the arms and legs using focused breaths and then relax and just let go. Be there for three minutes or more.

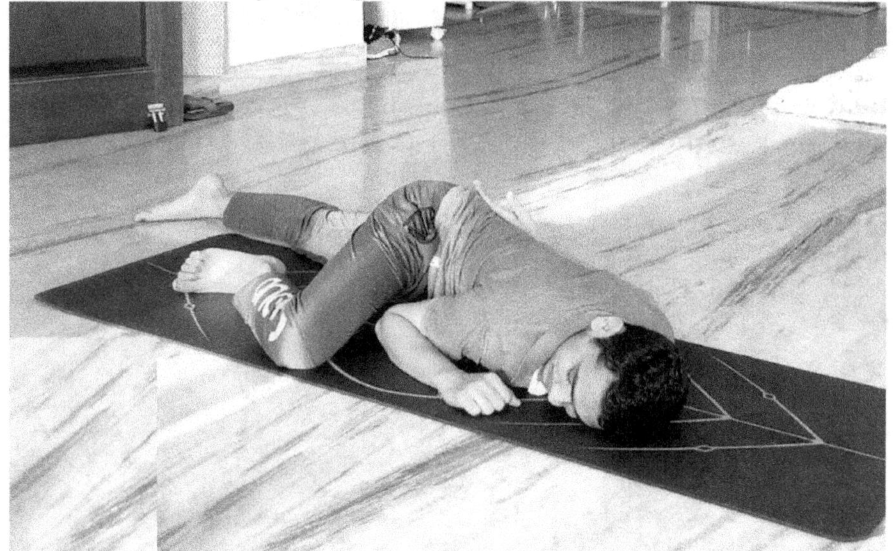

## Shavasana

Gently roll over to the back and rest in shavasana for a couple of minutes more. Make your breath very normal. Make your posture very limp. Relax deeply.

**Feel renewed, invigorated, refreshed, even more grateful**

Gently roll over to the right side, and slowly come to a sitting position, with the help of your arms and hands.

Stretch your legs out in the front and shake them a bit. Massage the knees and ankles.

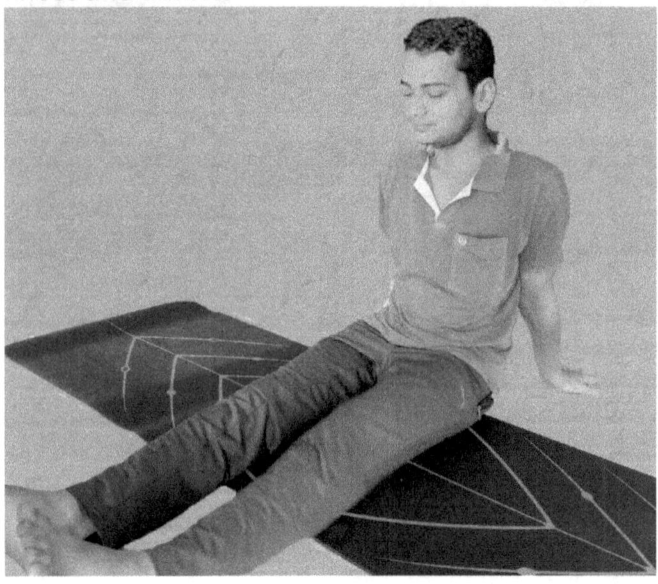

**Butterfly**

Feet together clasped by the hands. Start flapping the knees up and down, spine straight. Go full pace, then slow down and stop. Inhale and go back, exhale and bend forward to touch your forehead to the floor.

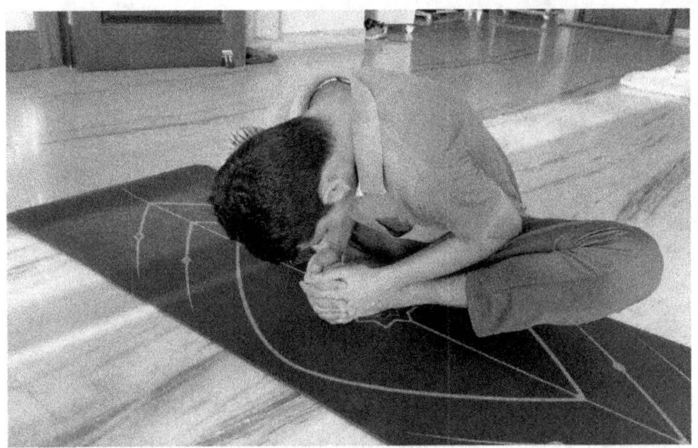

Release and flap your legs to evaporate any strain. Massage the knees and ankles.

CLOCK 54 minutes elapsed
**Paschimottanasana**

Sitting forward bend.

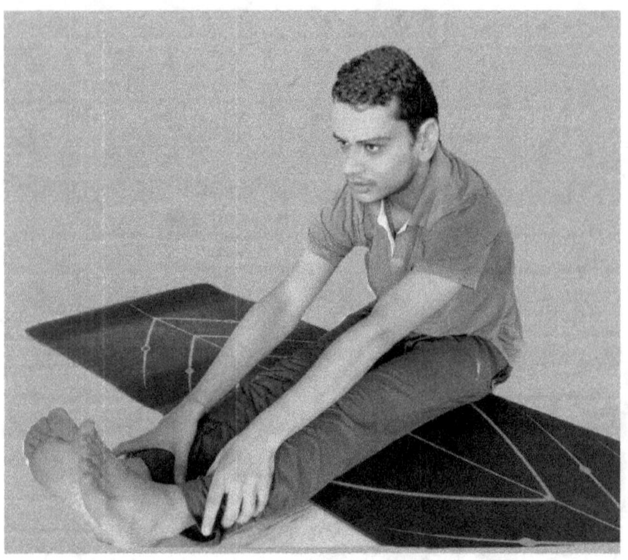

Feet together, arms go up and back as you inhale. Then exhale and bend forward from the waist, keeping the arms parallel to each other. Allow the outstretched hands to drop to touch the legs wherever you can. Bend more and inch your hands forward. Then take your head down, chest down. Hold for six good breaths.

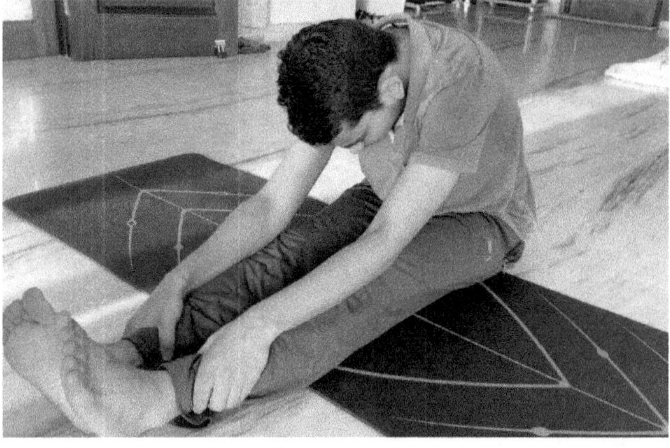

Inhale and slide your hands back on the legs and relax.

Sitting Sideways Spinal Twist

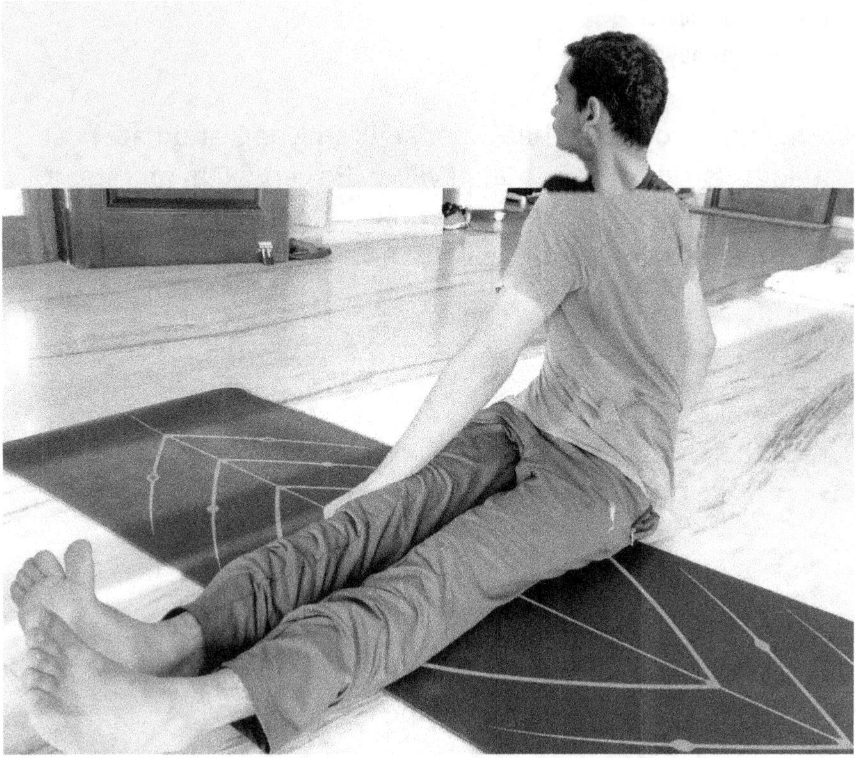

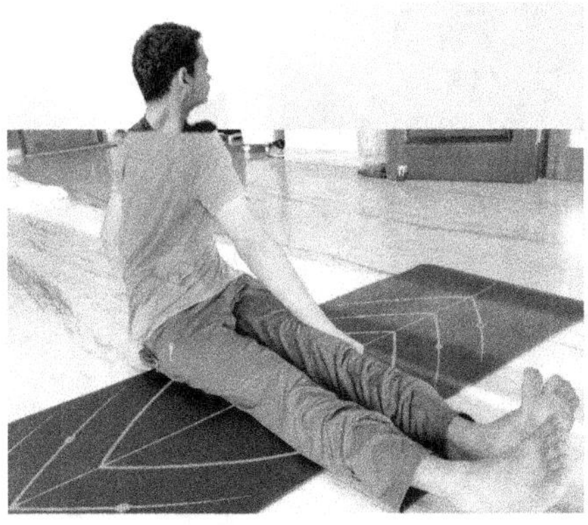

Left hand on floor near right knee. Right hand behind the back on the floor. Twist the torso and look back as much as you can. Take six good breaths.

Inhale, and as you exhale come to the center. Repeat the other side, look to the left.

**Nadi Shodan Pranayama**

Let us do three rounds of Nadi Shodan Pranayama alternate nostril breathing. Also known as Anulom Vilom. Be very silent and steady in the breath. Be aware of each incoming and outgoing breath. Make your breath long and smooth, and silent.


**Heart Center**

Locating the Sternum Marma Point, and tapping there.

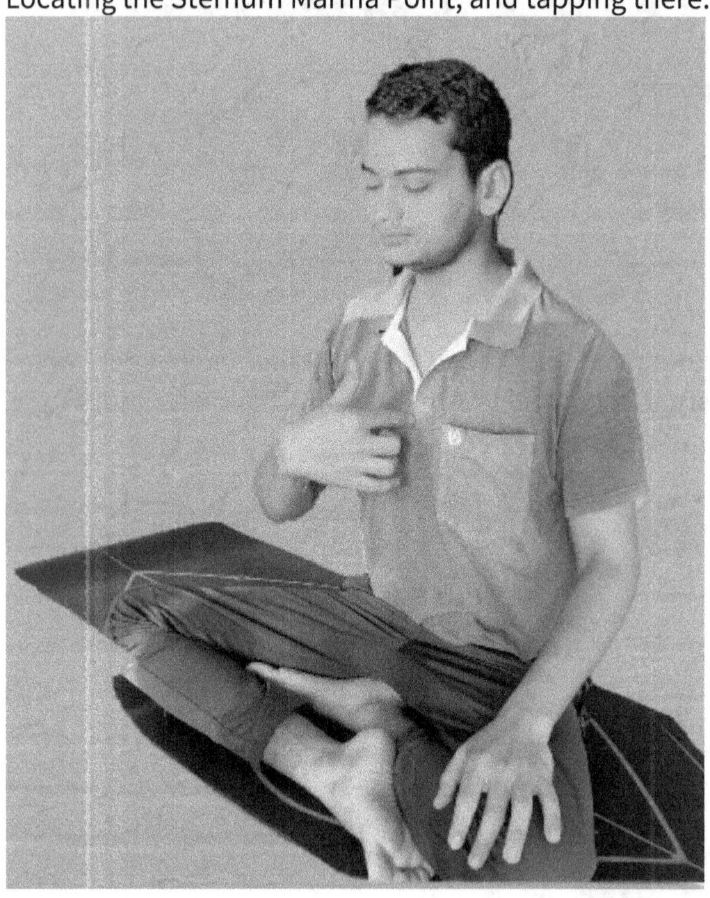

Flow of Prana or Consciousness
Now sit at ease. Close the eyes. Allow the mind to come to the present moment. Let go of excess thoughts. Do not chase any.

Palms in Dhyana Mudra, left palm below the right palm, placed at the midline loosely.

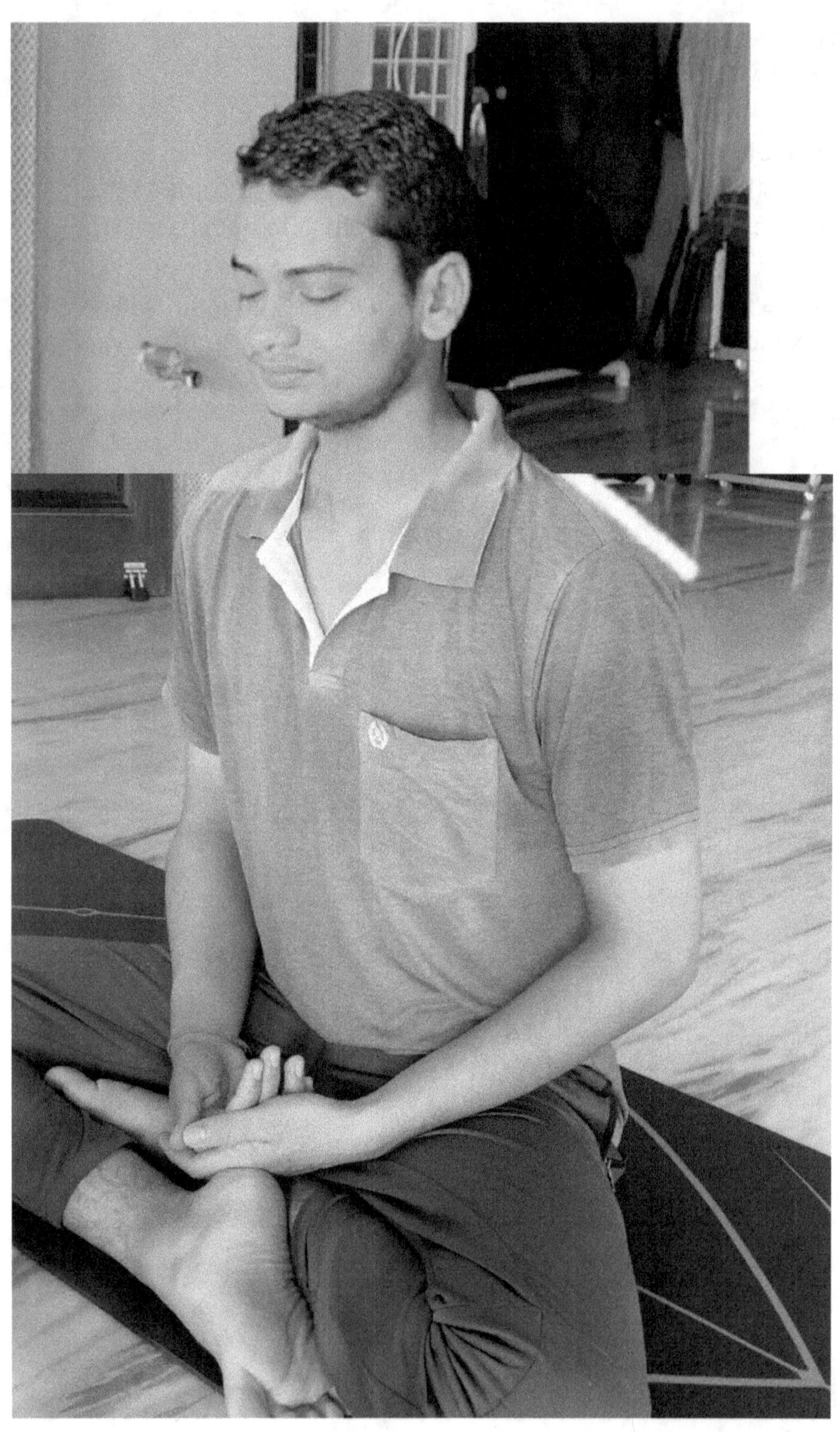

Keep your mind very soft, very relaxed.

Take your attention to the center of the chest, at the sternum. Do
not be too precise in your reasoning, let your body guide you.
Whatever point you imagine, it's okay.

Gather your mind at this point.
Penetrate the point, go deep inside the chest.
Allow the mind to travel slowly inside the chest, until you reach the
spine. Might feel some sensation along the spine too. Be with it.

This is the Anāhata Chakra (literally, an āhata = un struck).
The heart center.

As you inhale, imagine you are drawing your breath from the heart
center on the spine to the sternum. As you exhale, you are pushing
your breath out from the spine.

INHALE = breath moves from SPINE to STERNUM
EXHALE = push the breath out from the Spinal point.

You are piercing the Anāhata Chakra with each breath.
Keep your mind soft.

Let your breath polish your chest.
Polish the anāhata chakra, heart center.

Deep breath in, exhale, release your attention from the breath,
bring it back to the chest. Just be with yourself.
Release your mind, let it go. Be at rest.

Take a deep breath in and exhale completely.

Bring your hands in Namaste, folded prayerful position. Feel a love
for yourself, the creation, and your family.

Rub you palms together, place them on the eyes, and gently open your eyes with a smile.

10-minute Meditation finishes
Get up, the session is done.

# Asana Sequence

| | |
|---|---|
| 1. Warm Up = *power walk*<br>CLOCK 00:00 | 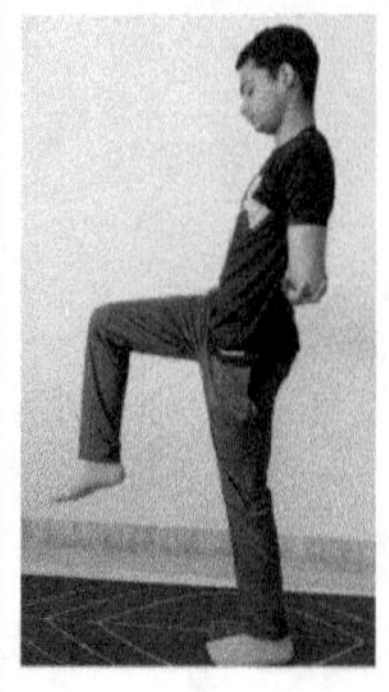 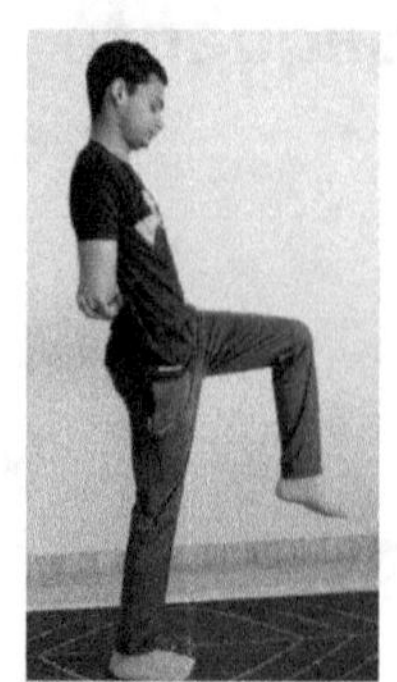 |
| *2.* Prayer = *Om Chant*<br>CLOCK 00:05 | 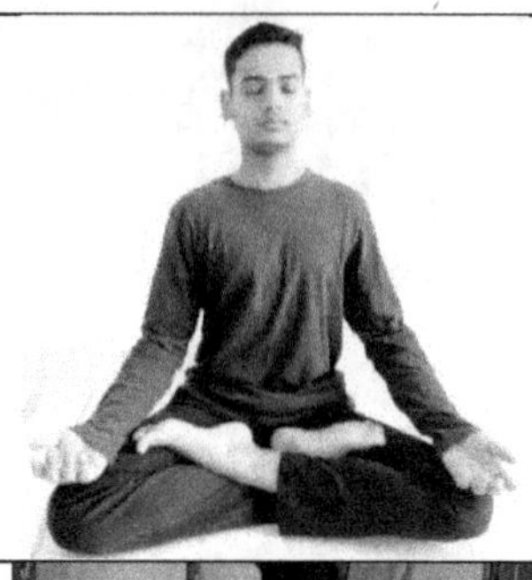 |
| 3. Pranayama = *bhastrika*<br>CLOCK 00:08 | |
| 4. Pelvic Rotations = *deha chankramana*<br>CLOCK 00:11 | 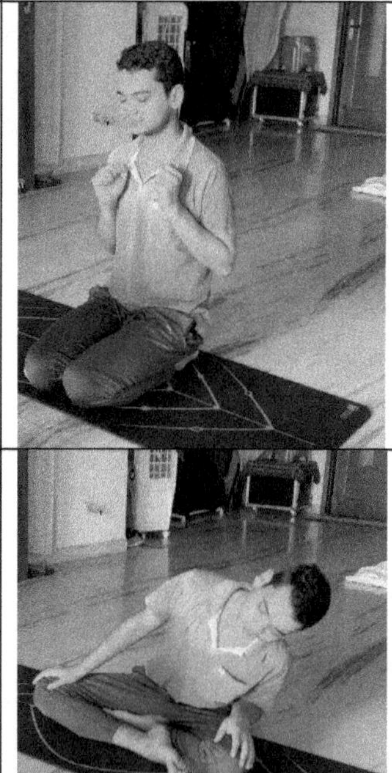 |

| 5.  Bandha Locks<br>**CLOCK 00:13** | 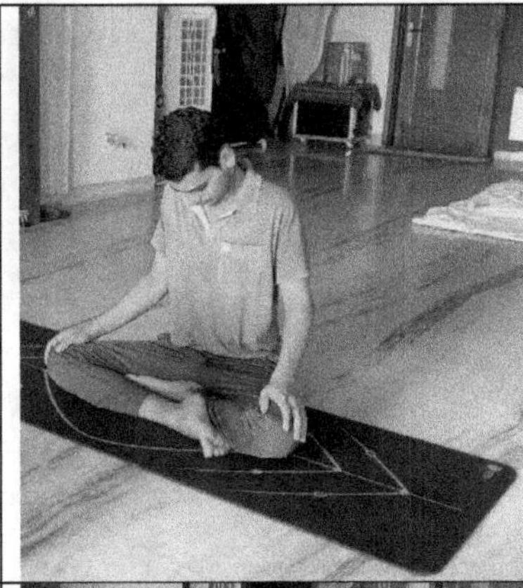 |
| 6.  Arm Movement<br>**CLOCK 00:14** | 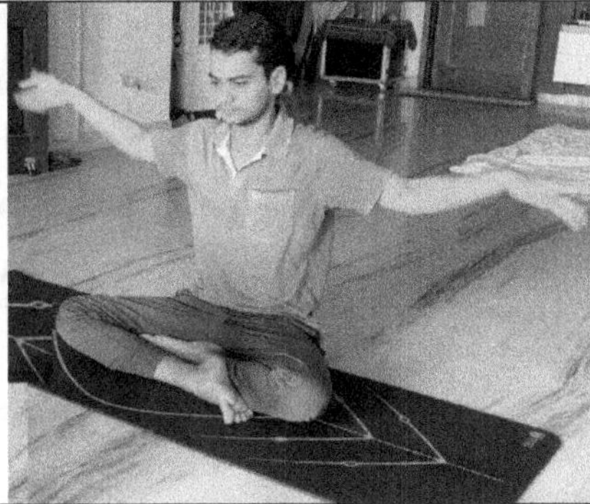 |
| 7.  Jogging with Dance<br>**CLOCK 00:16** | 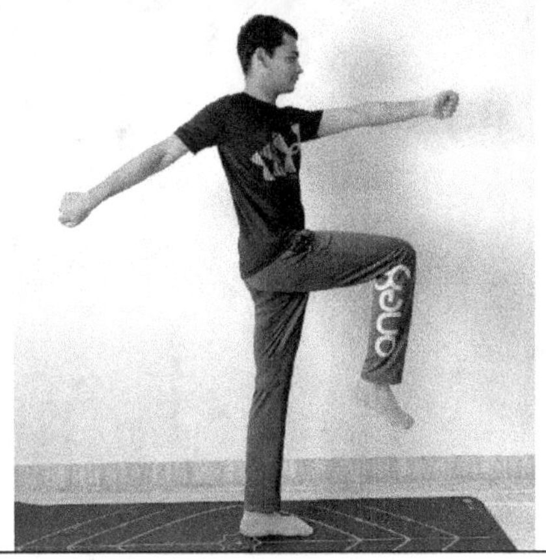 |

| 8. Hum Sound<br>CLOCK 00:19 | 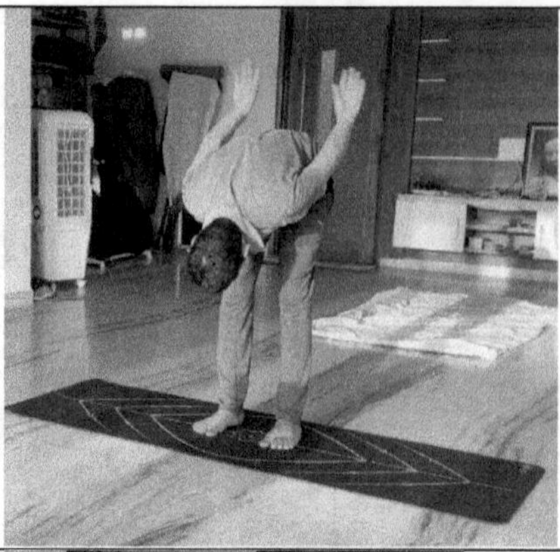 |
| 9. Torso Bends<br>CLOCK 00:21 | 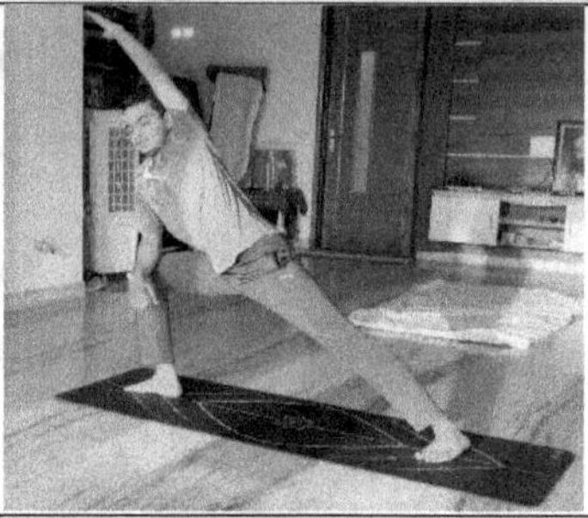 |
| 10. Warrior I<br>CLOCK 00:23 | 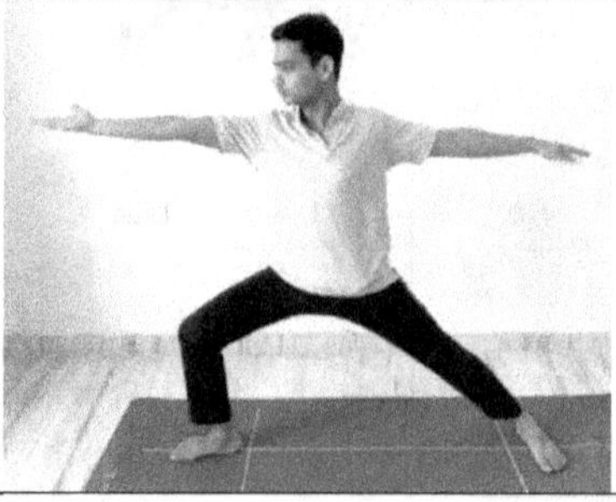 |
| 11. Warrior II<br>CLOCK 00:25 | 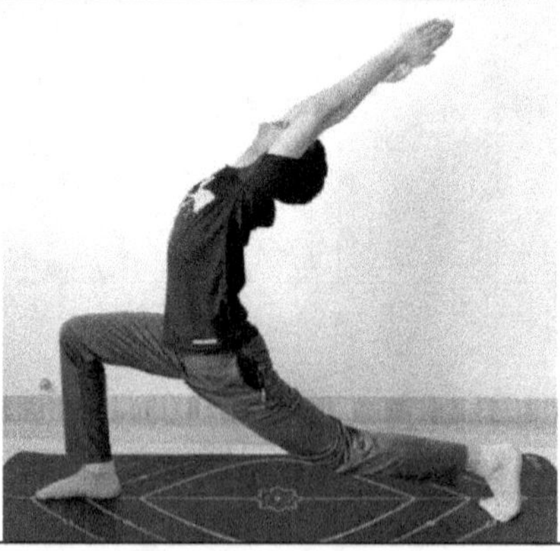 |

| | |
|---|---|
| 12. Triangle =<br>*trikonasana*<br>CLOCK 00:27 | 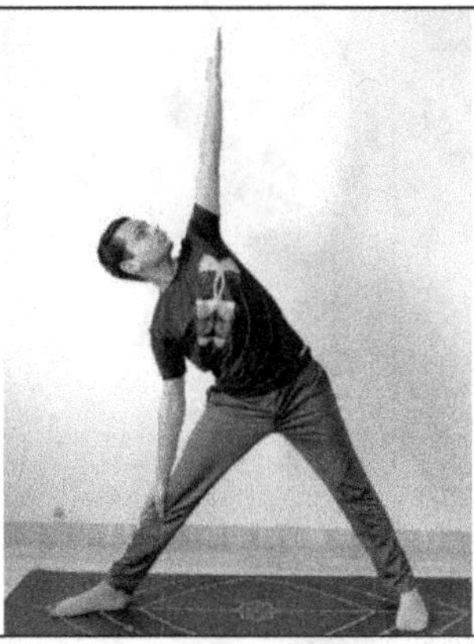 |
| 13. Back Bend =<br>*pristha pranati*<br>CLOCK 00:28 | 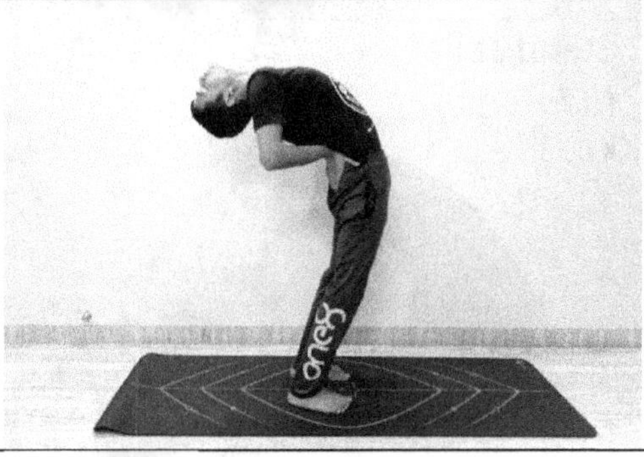 |
| 14. Forward Bend<br>= *pada*<br>*hastāsana*<br>CLOCK 00:29 | 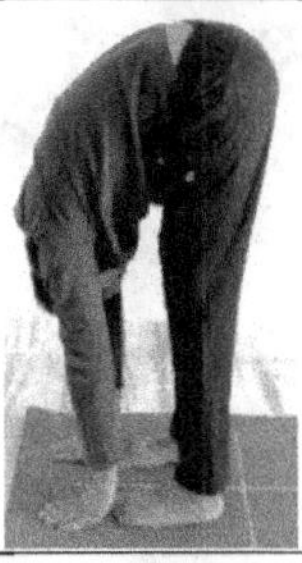 |
| *15.* Chair = *utkat*<br>*āsana*<br>CLOCK 00:30 | 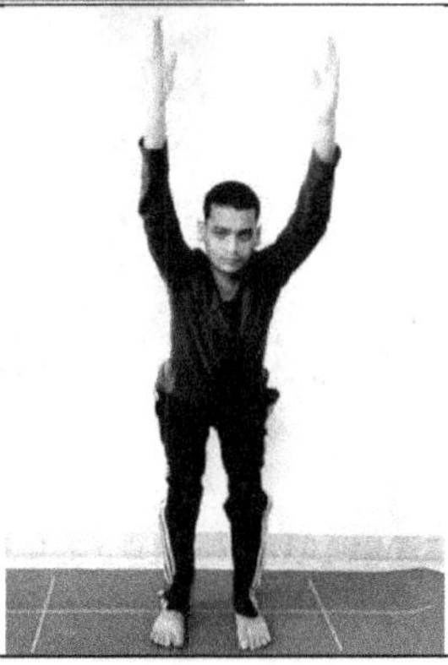 |

| | |
|---|---|
| **16. Up and Back =** *uttana hastāsana* <br> CLOCK 00:31 | 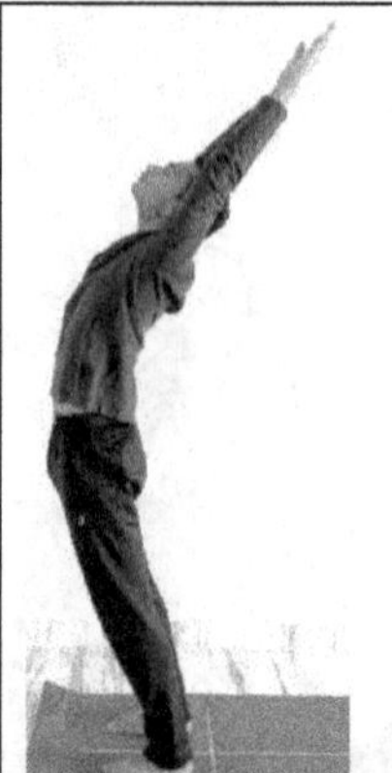 |
| **17. Stand Tall =** *tadasana* <br> CLOCK 00:32 | 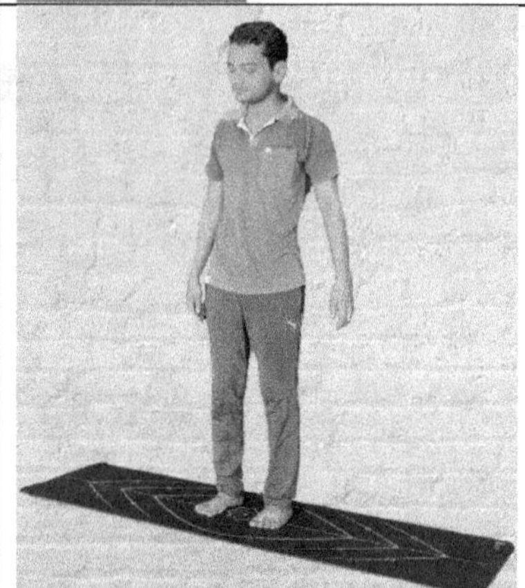 |
| **18. Twist Right =** *kati chakra āsana* <br> CLOCK 00:34 <br><br> And twist left | 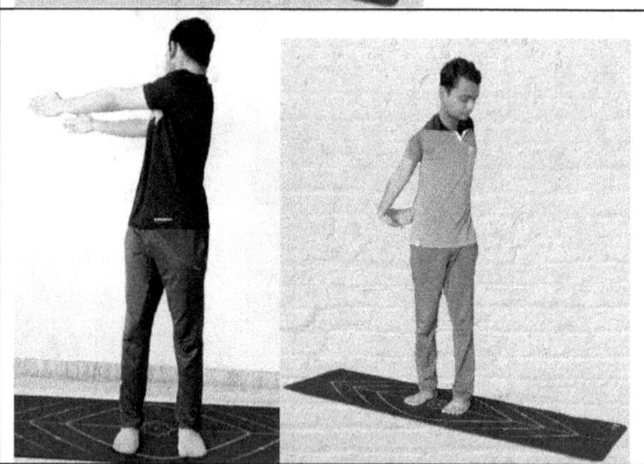 |

| 19. Roll Shoulders<br>CLOCK 00:35 | 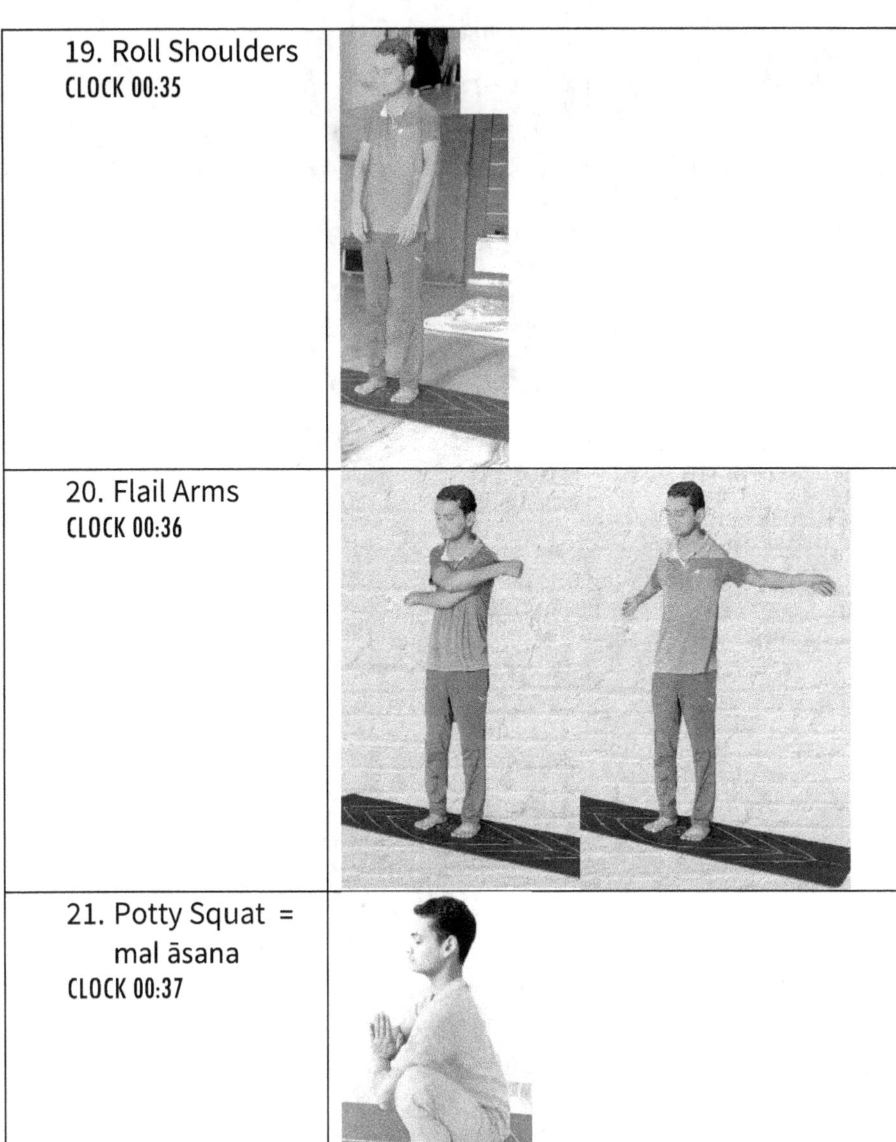 |
| 20. Flail Arms<br>CLOCK 00:36 | |
| 21. Potty Squat =<br>mal āsana<br>CLOCK 00:37 | |

| 22. Ha! Sound<br>CLOCK 00:38 | 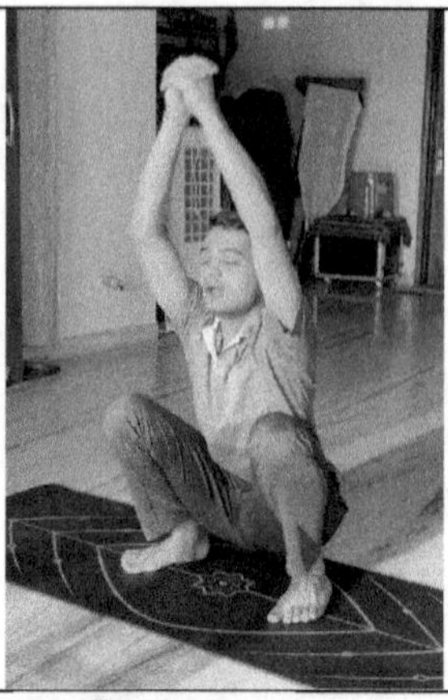 |
| 23. Cow Face =<br>*gomukhasana*<br>CLOCK 00:39 | 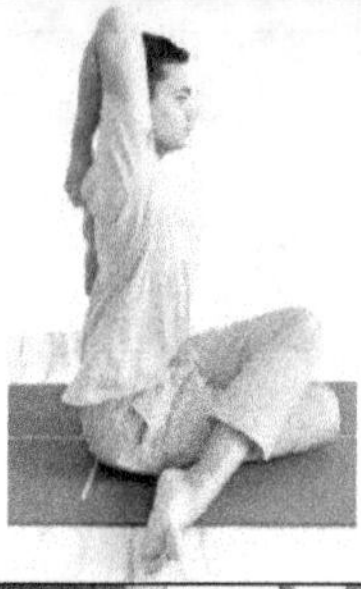 |
| 24. Lowered Plank<br>CLOCK 00:40 | 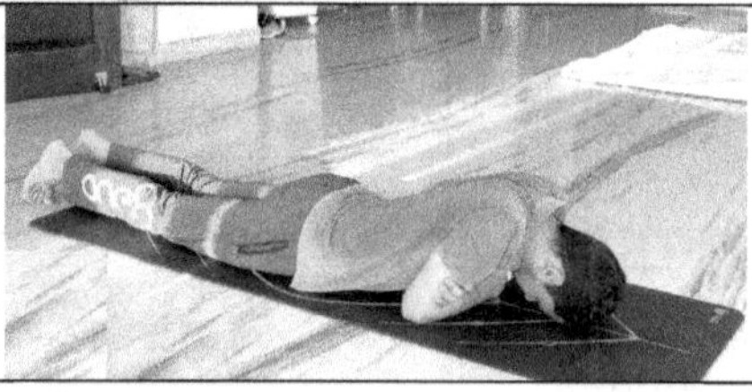 |
| 25. Plank =<br>*caturanga*<br>*dandāsana*<br>CLOCK 00:41 | 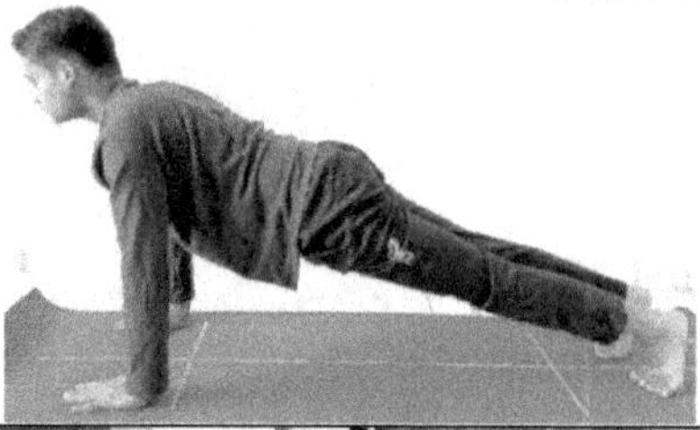 |
| 26. Elbow Plank<br>CLOCK 00:42 | 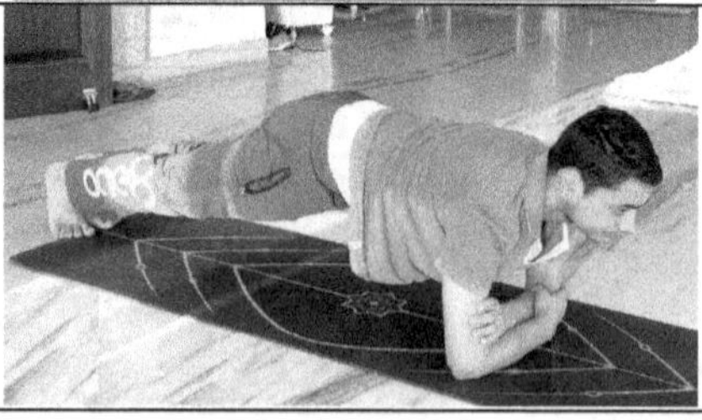 |

| | |
|---|---|
| **27. Cobra =** *bhujangāsana* CLOCK 00:43<br><br>or sphinx pose | |
| **28. Relax =** *makarāsana* CLOCK 00:44 | |
| **29. Bow =** *dhanurāsana* CLOCK 00:45 | |
| **30. Comfort Relax =** *suptvishnuāsana* CLOCK 00:46 | |
| **31. Corpse =** shavasana CLOCK 00:47 | |
| **32. Roll to Right =** shavasana CLOCK 00:52 | |

| | |
|---|---|
| 33. Butterfly = <br> *titliāsana* <br> CLOCK 00:53 | 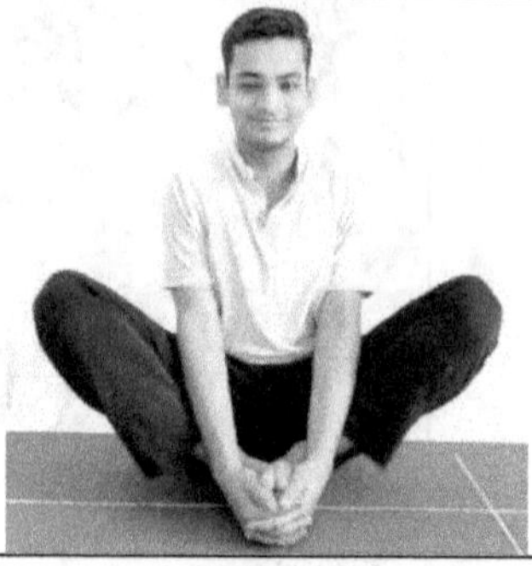 |
| 34. Sitting forward bend = <br> paschimottāsana <br> CLOCK 00:54 | 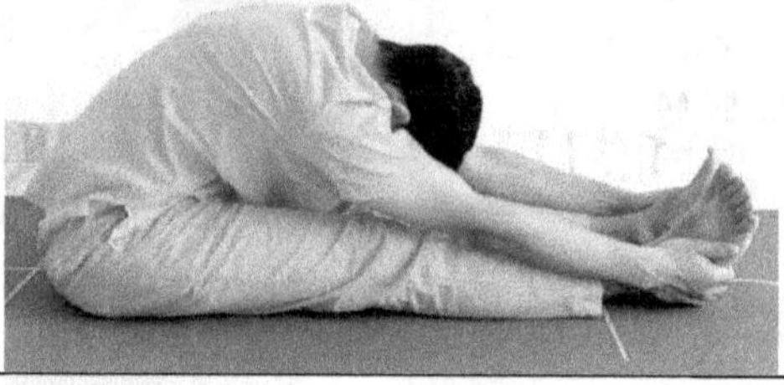 |
| 35. Sitting sideways twist <br> CLOCK 00:55 | 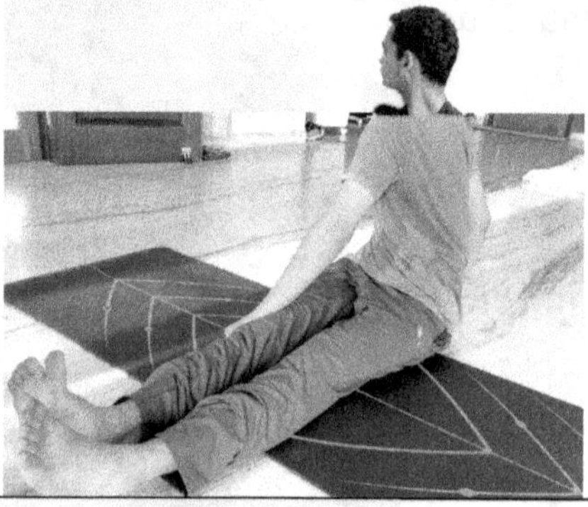 |
| 36. Alternate Nostril Breathing = <br> *nadi shodhan pranayama* <br> CLOCK 00:56 | 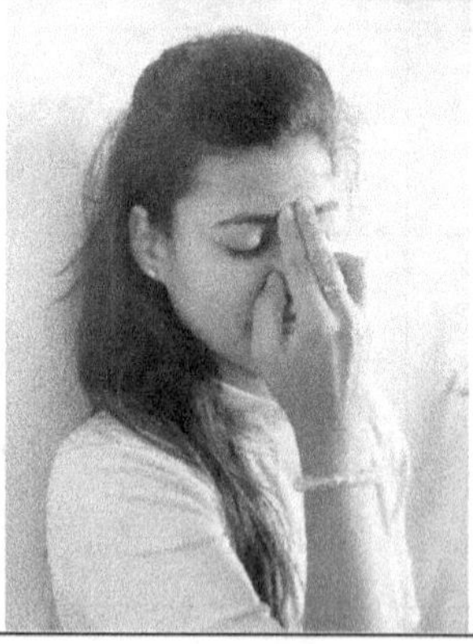 |

| 37. Heart Center =<br>*anahata chakra*<br>CLOCK 00:58 | 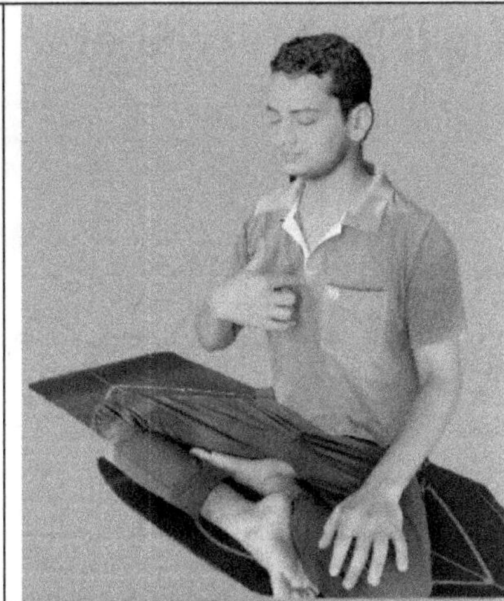 |
| 38. Final<br>  Meditation<br>  with Dhyana<br>  Mudra<br>CLOCK 01:00 | 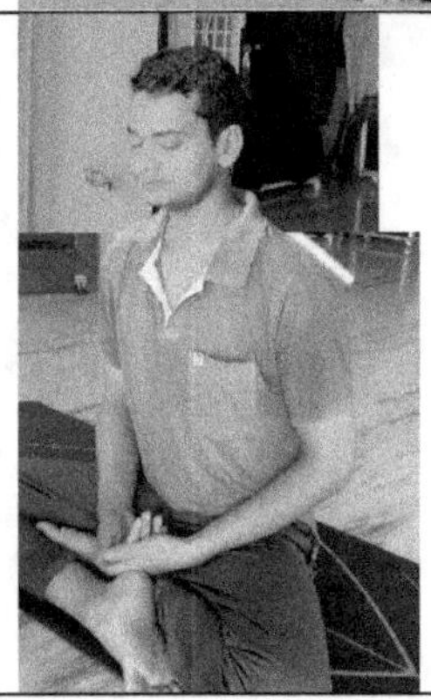 |

# Asana Self-Explanatory Shots

## 1. Warm Ups and Cool Down = **CLOCK HH:MM 00:00**

power brain yoga sit-ups, power walk

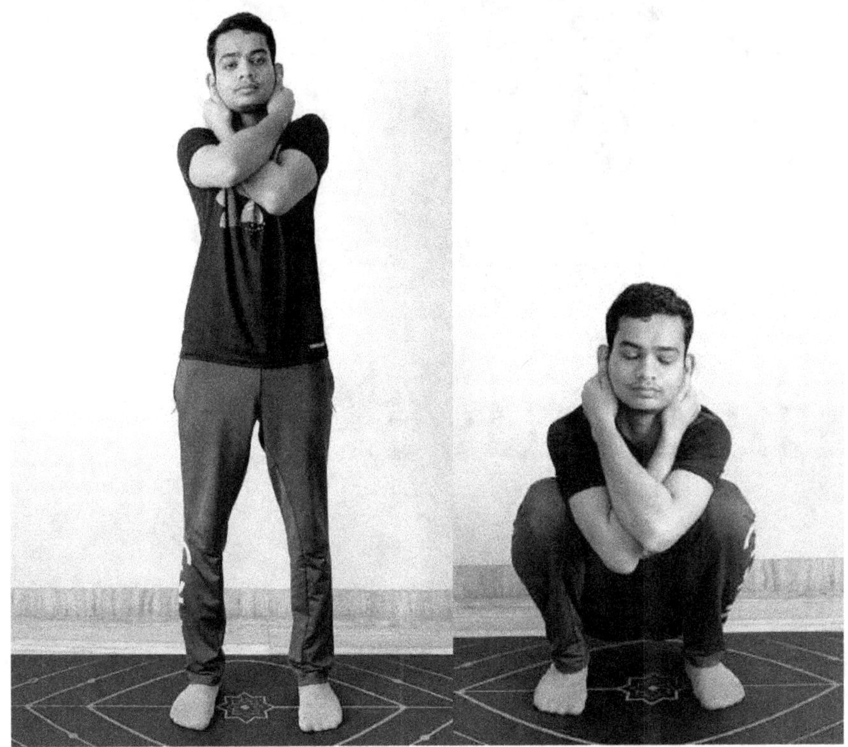

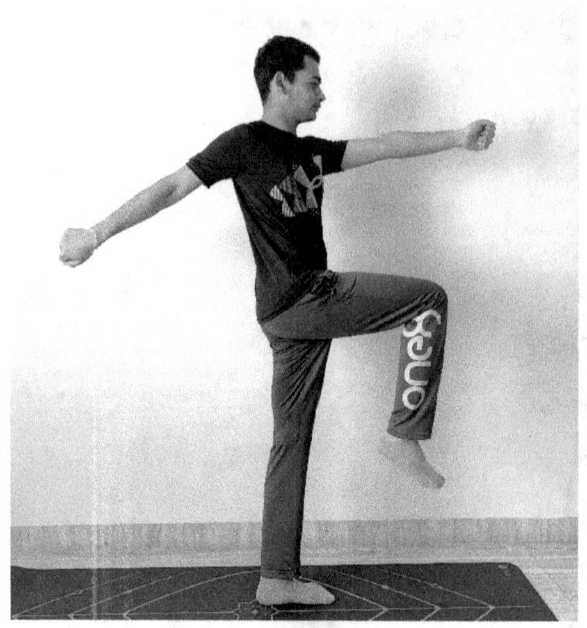

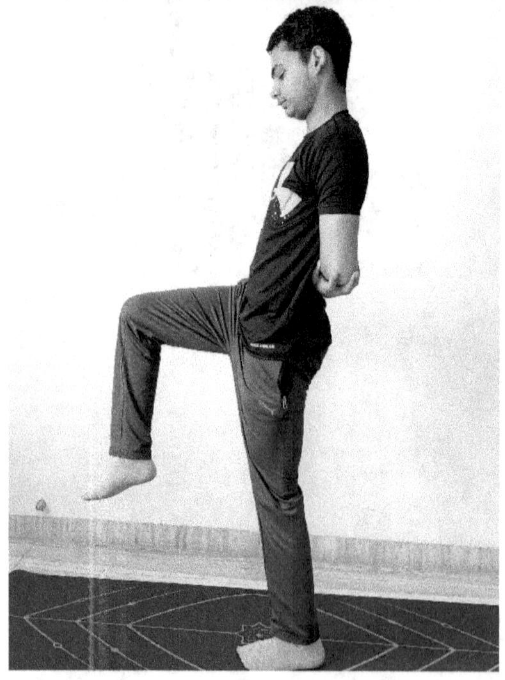

2. Prayer = **CLOCK 00:05**

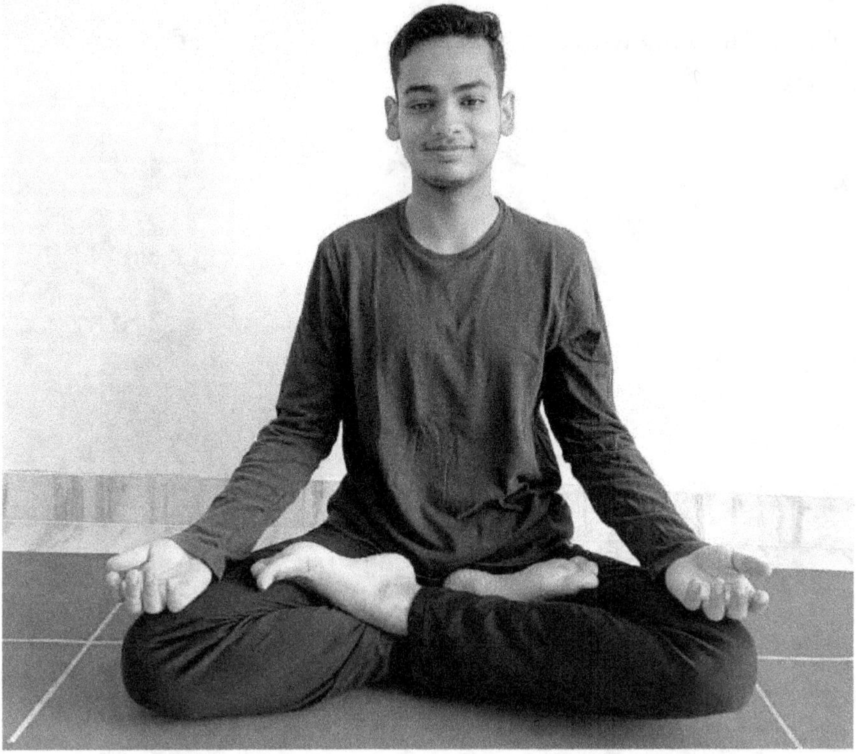

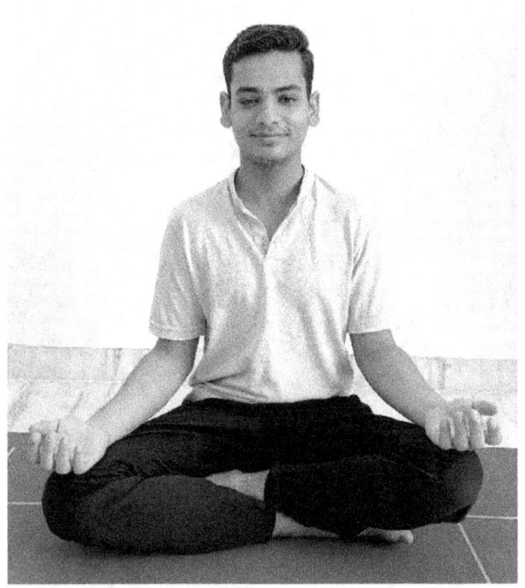

Be with yourself. Take a few deep breaths. Chant Om thrice.

## 3. Pranayama Bhastrika = **CLOCK 00:08**

Bellows Breathing with arm and hand movements. Sitting in Vajrasana.

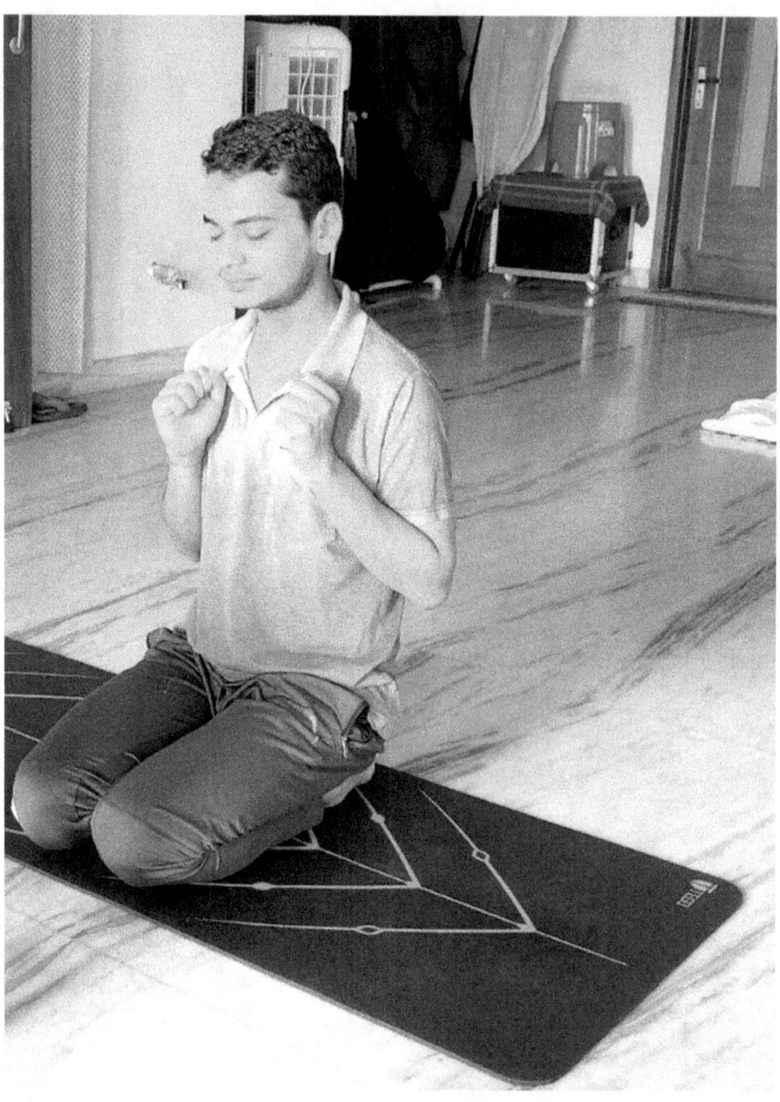

## 4. Pelvic Rotation = **CLOCK 00:11**
deha chankramana

A      B

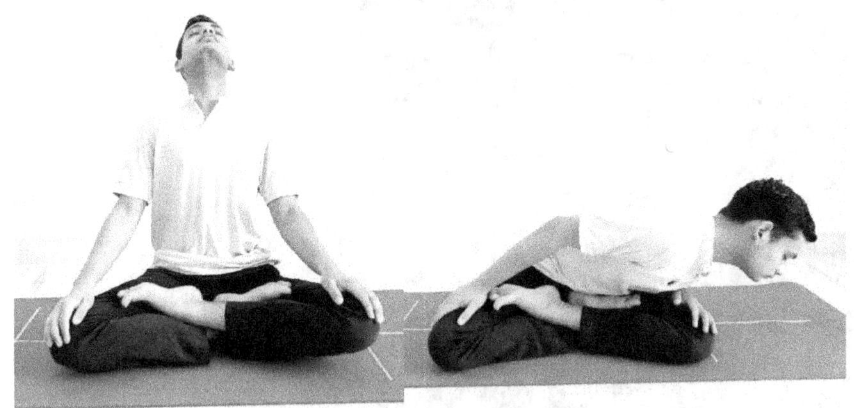

6 rounds Clockwise rotation, followed by anticlockwise 6 rounds.

C      D

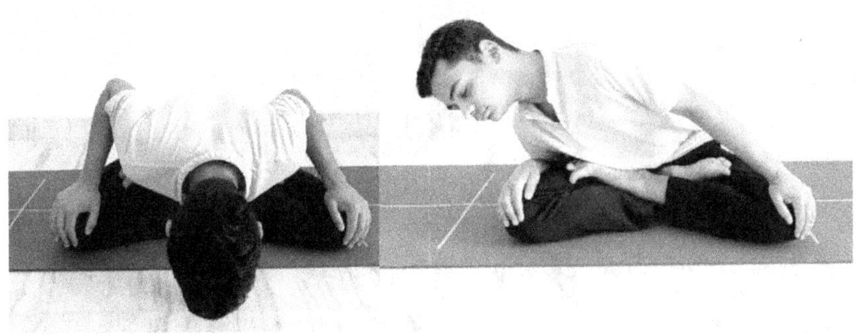

## 5. Bandha Locks = **CLOCK 00:13**

moolbandh and jalandhar bandh

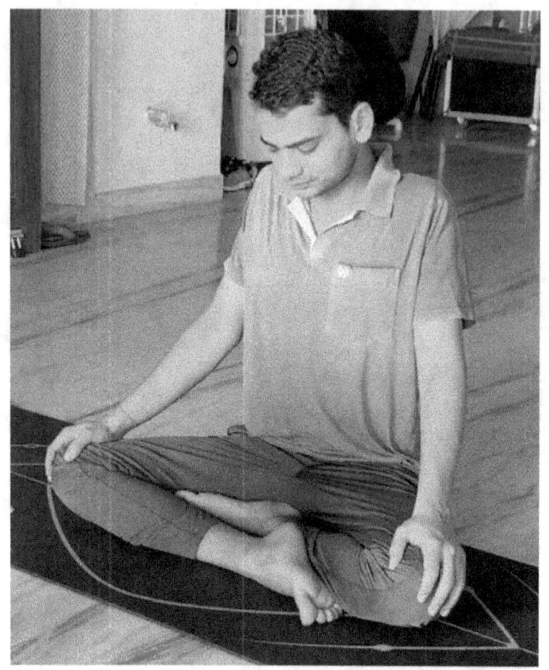

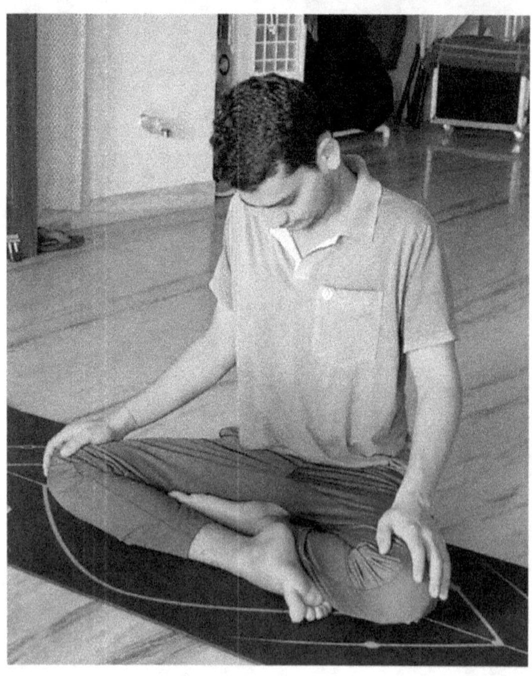

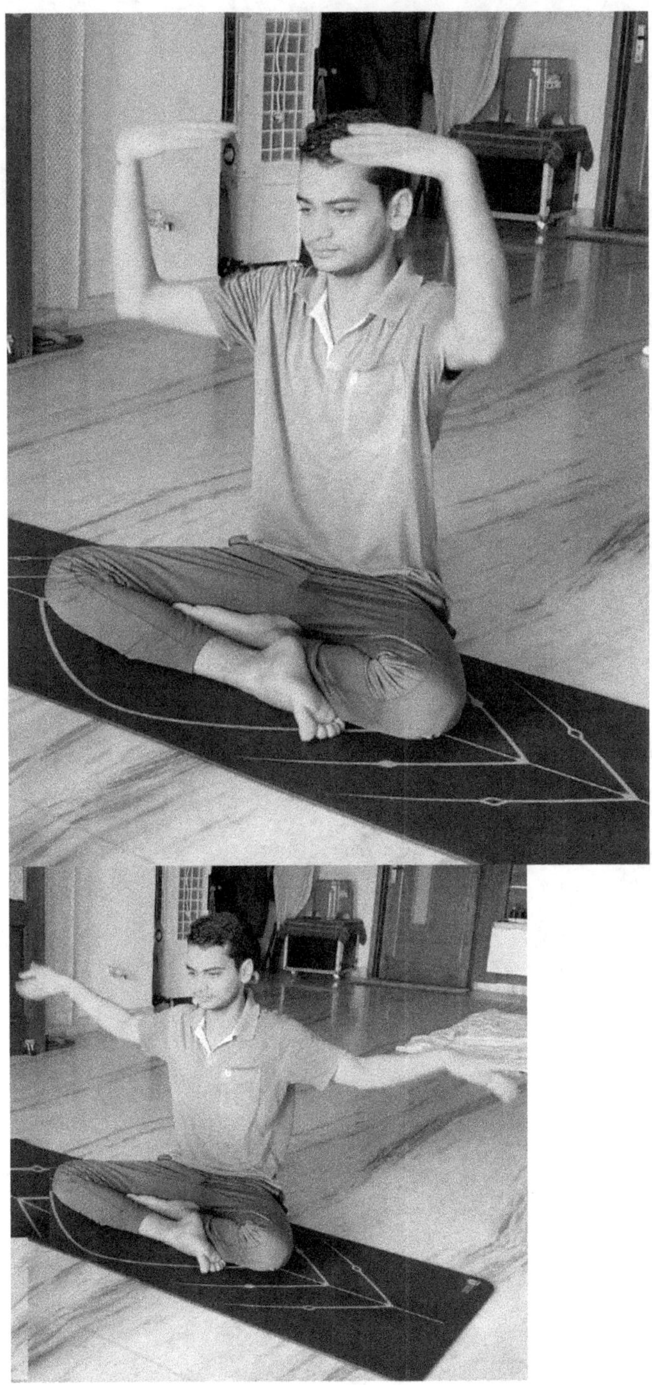

# 7. Jogging and freestyle Dance = **CLOCK 00:16**

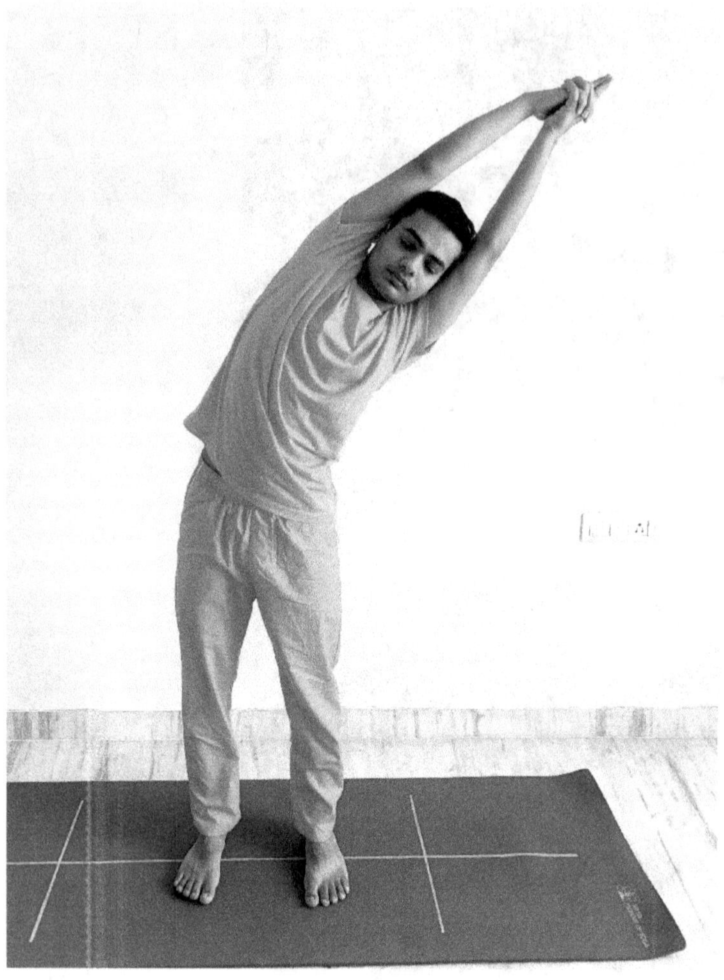

# 8. "Hum" Sound Loud = **CLOCK 00:19**

Stand straight and tall. Abdomen tight, pulled in, hips engaged. Go back in uttana hasta asana, breathe in, then exhal and bend forward letting go of the arms in a loud "Hum" sound. Do this thrice.

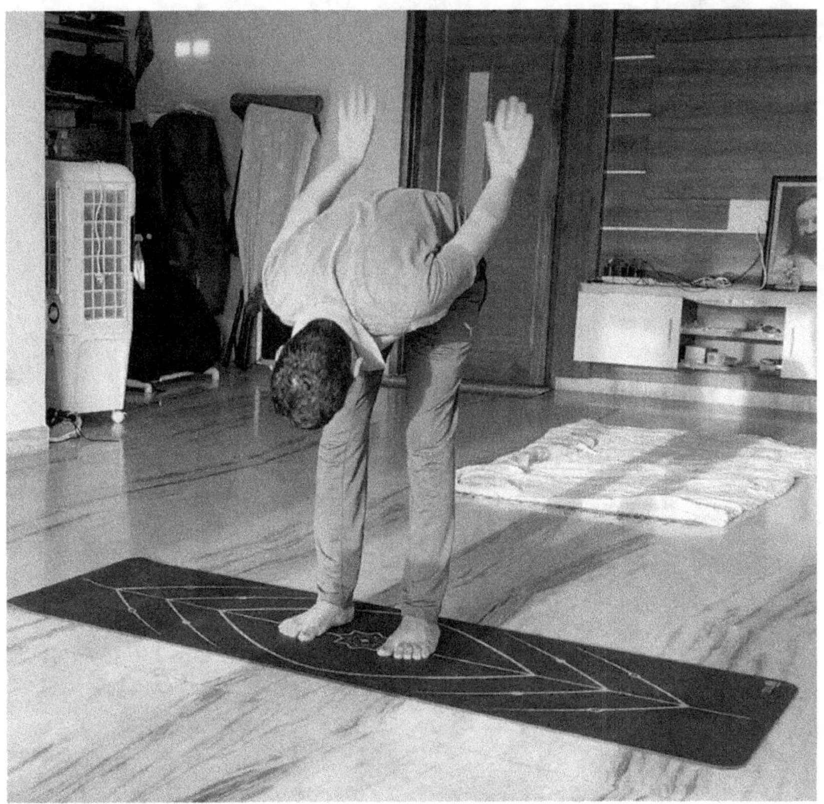

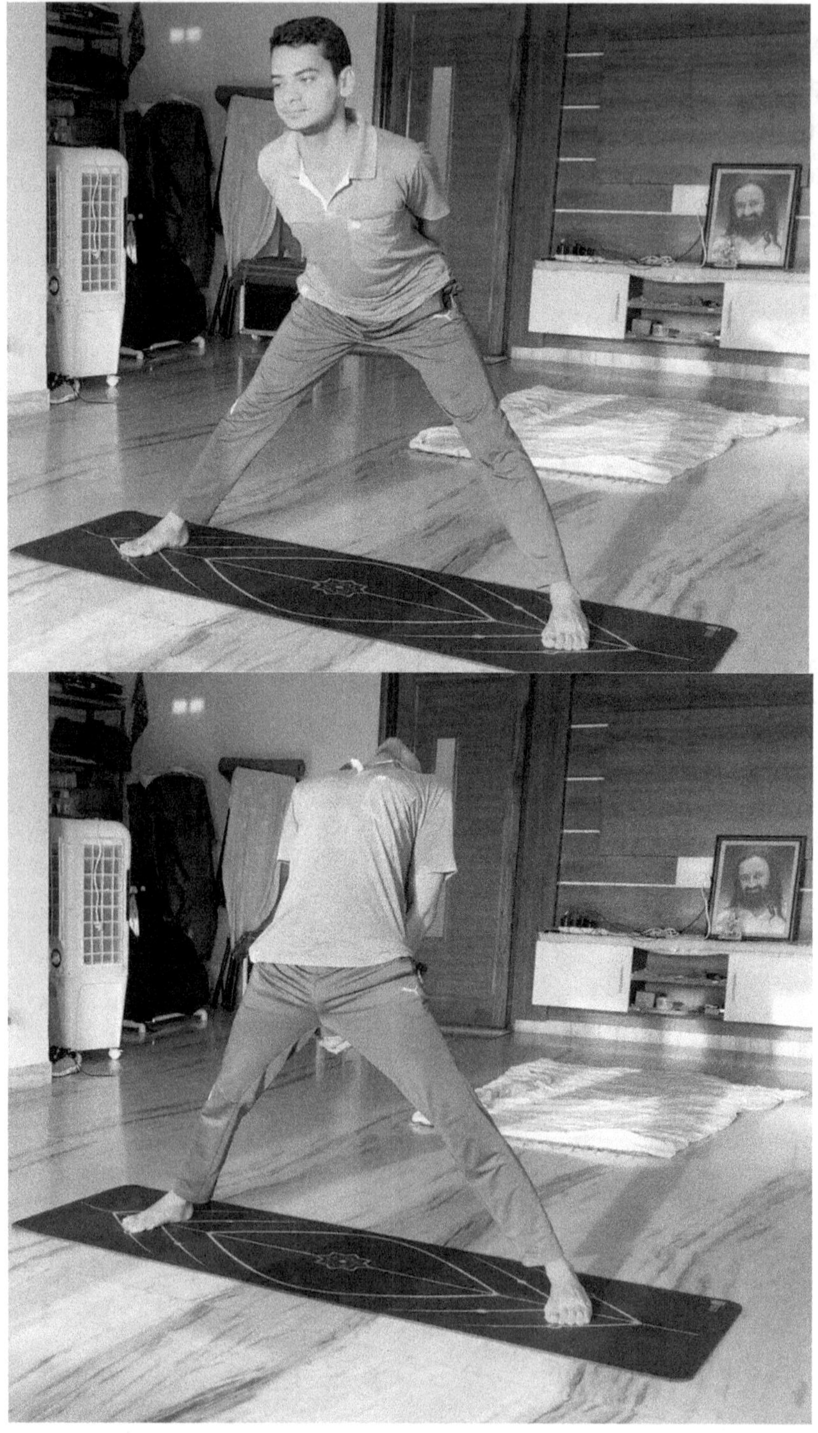

# 10. Warrior I = **CLOCK 00:23**
Virbhadrasana

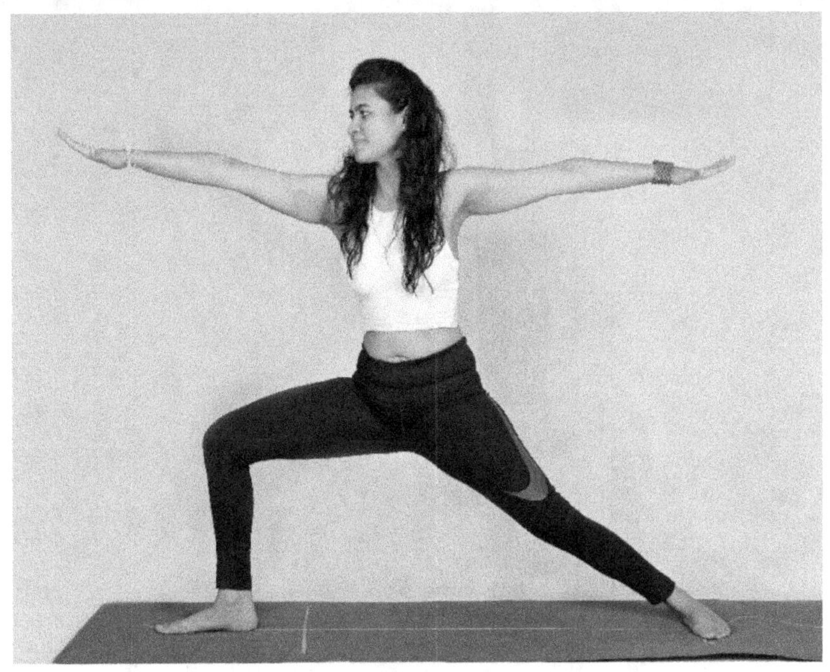

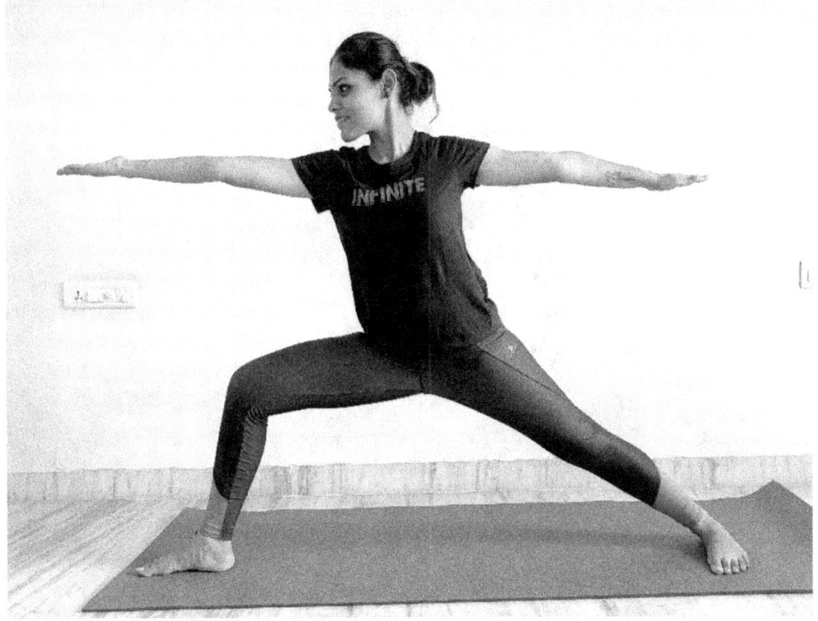

## 11. Warrior II = **CLOCK 00:25**

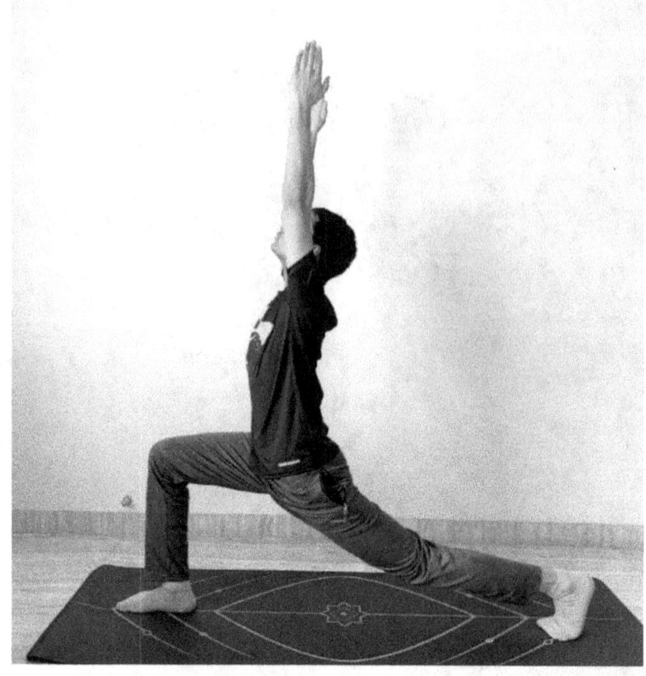

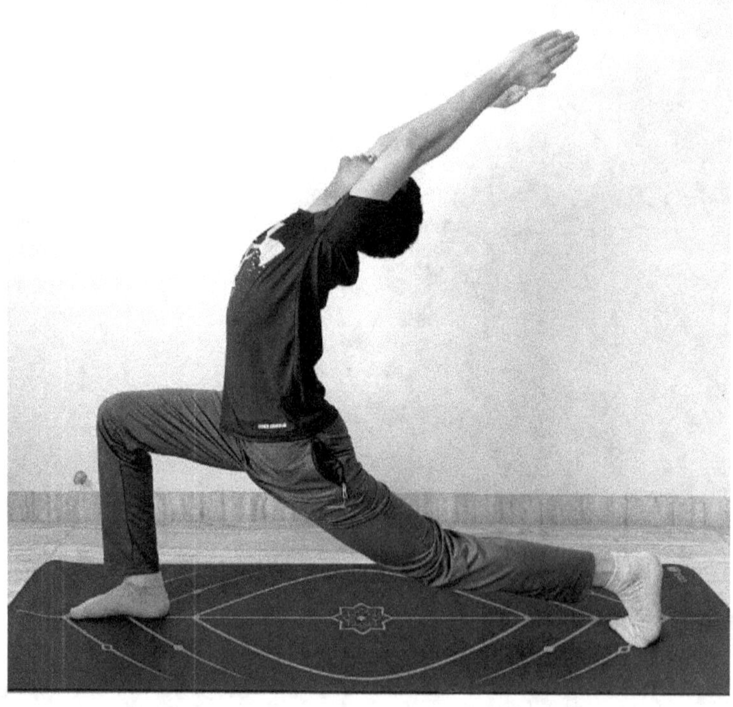

# 12. Triangle = **CLOCK 00:27**
Trikonasana

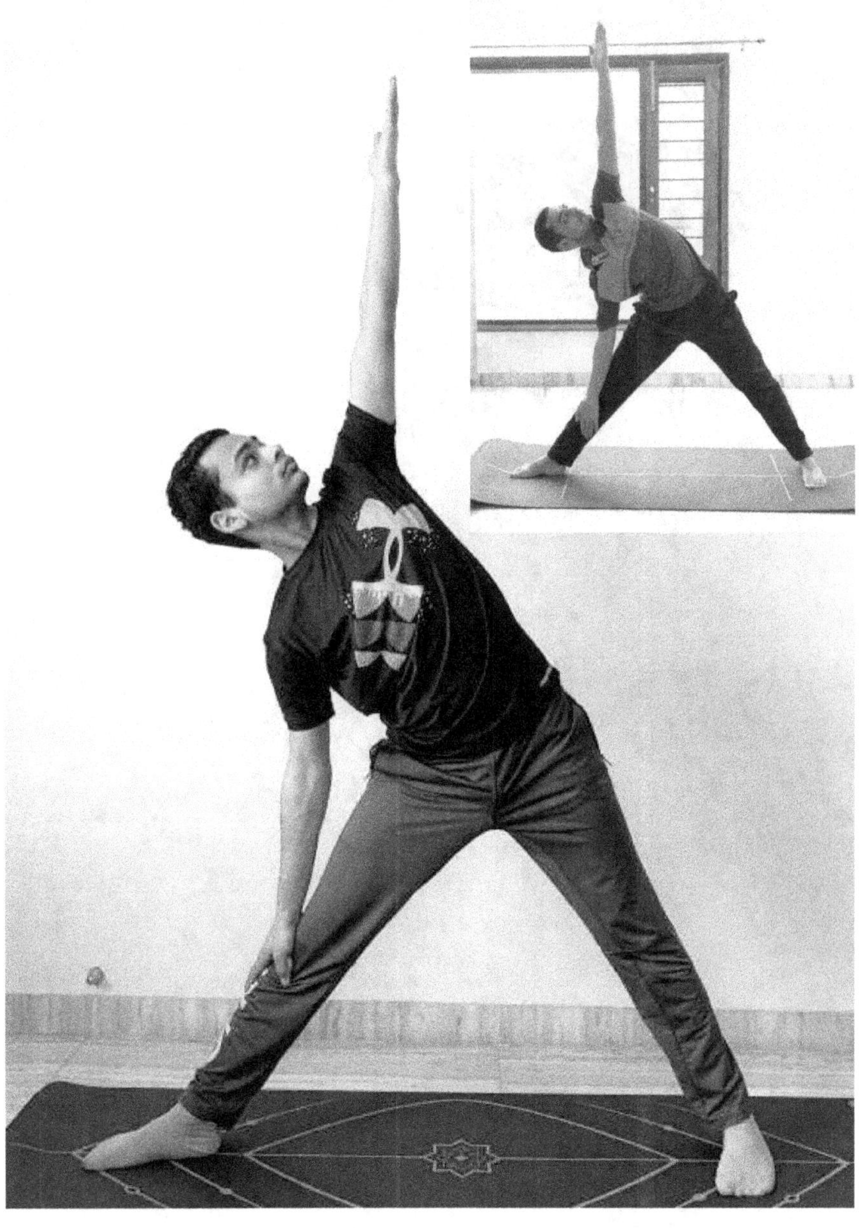

# 13. Back Bend = **CLOCK 00:28**

pristha pranati asana

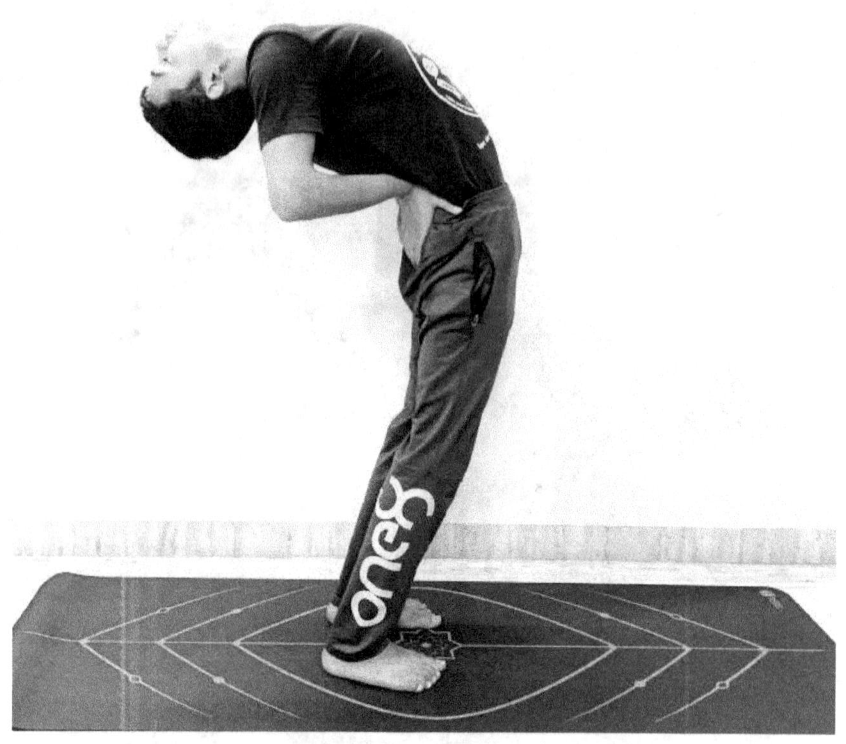

## 14. Forward Bend = **CLOCK 00:29**
pada hastasana

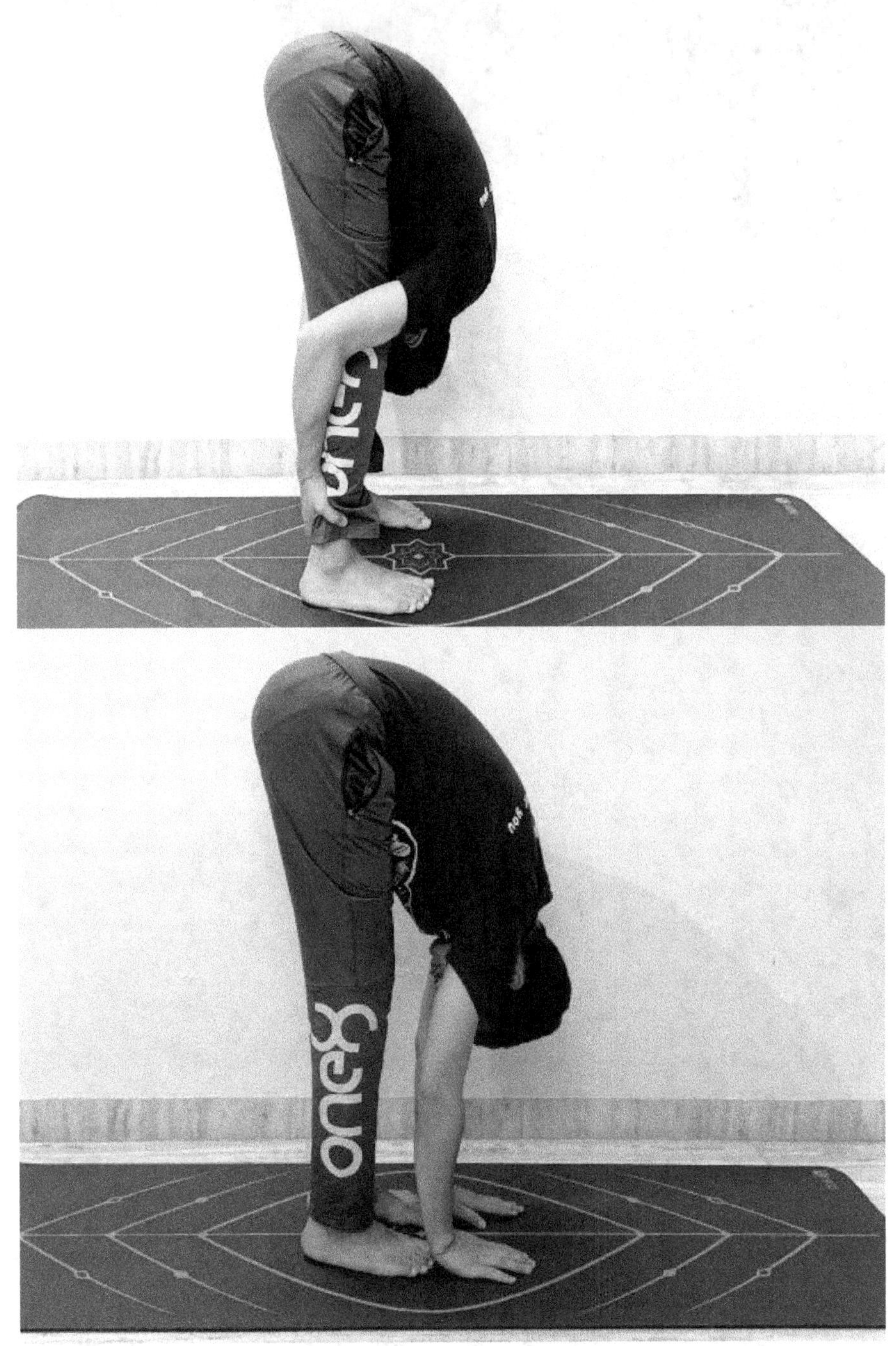

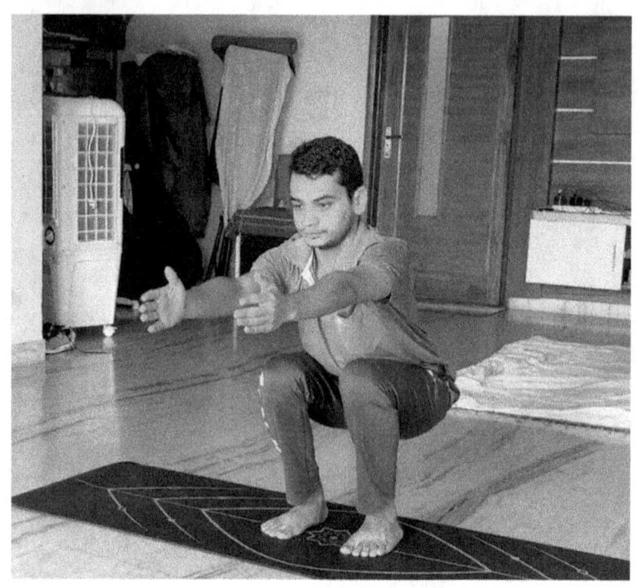

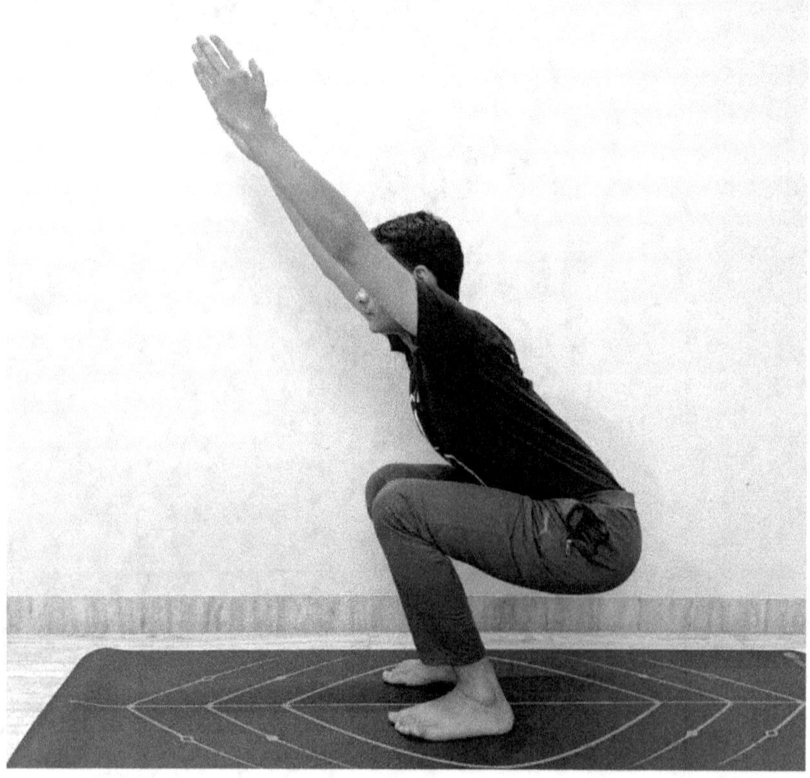

# 16. Up and Back = **CLOCK 00:31**
hasta uttanasana

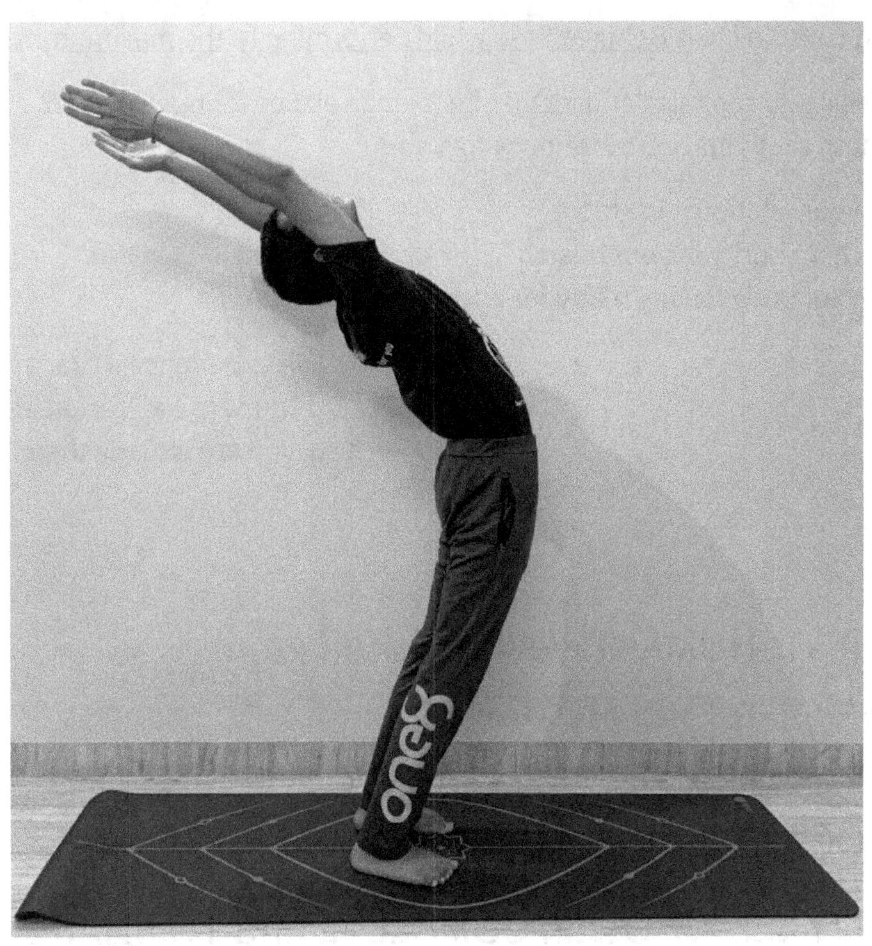

## Honoring the Practice

To covet in life is <u>Being at Ease while performing to the maximum</u>.

See if you can relax and let go after a quarrel. See for how long do these thoughts and emotions nag you…

Is your relationship stable?
Is there purity in your heart?
Is your body feeling ready for anything?

Do you experience a Grace?
Do you sense a Presence?
If so, you are already there.

This is HUMANITY's cherished goal.
Being in THIS MOMENT.

YOGA IS SIMPLY TO GET HERE.

TO FEEL WHOLE n COMPLETE and TO SHARE.

## 17. Stand Tall = **CLOCK 00:32**
tadasana

Take a deep breath in and become aware of the entire cosmos and willingly respond with each particle. Let the microcosm and the macrocosm become one and dissolve into the infinite.

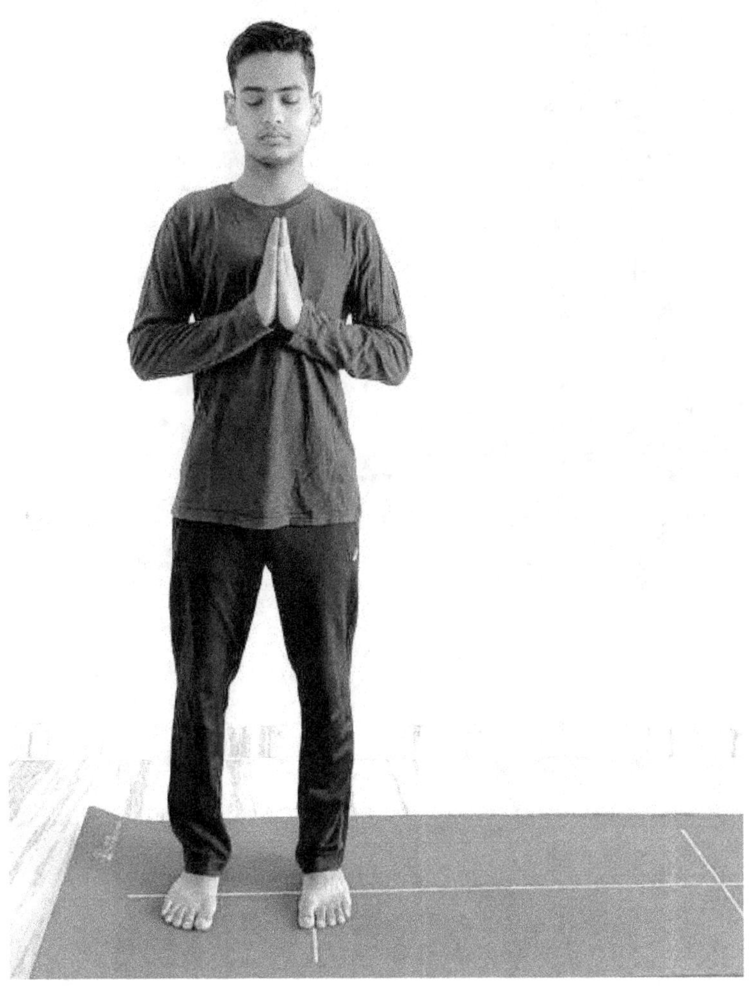

# 18. Twist along Transverse Axis Plane = **CLOCK 00:34**
katichakrasana

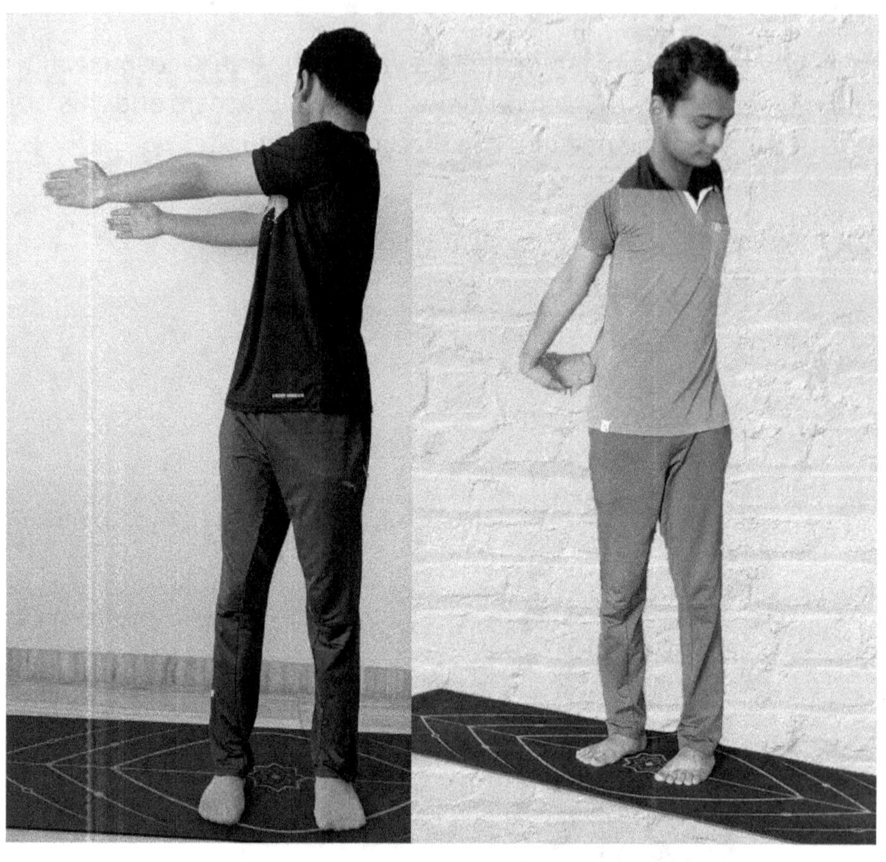

skandha chankramana

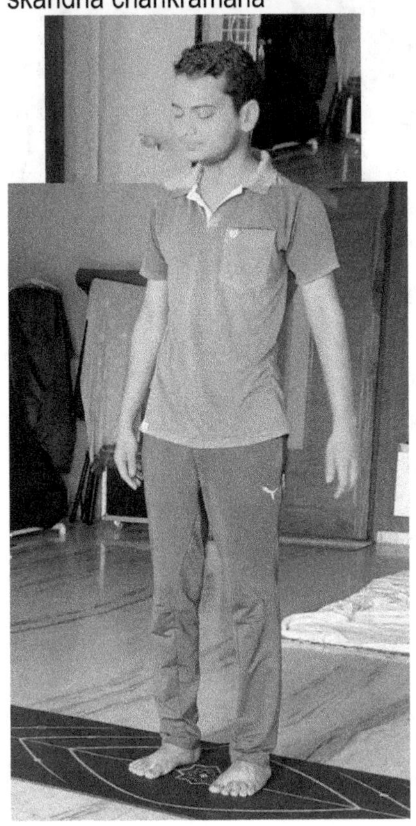 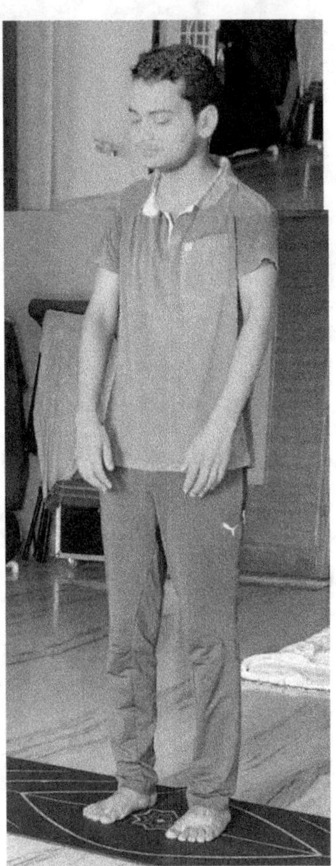

## 20. Arms Flail = **CLOCK 00:36**

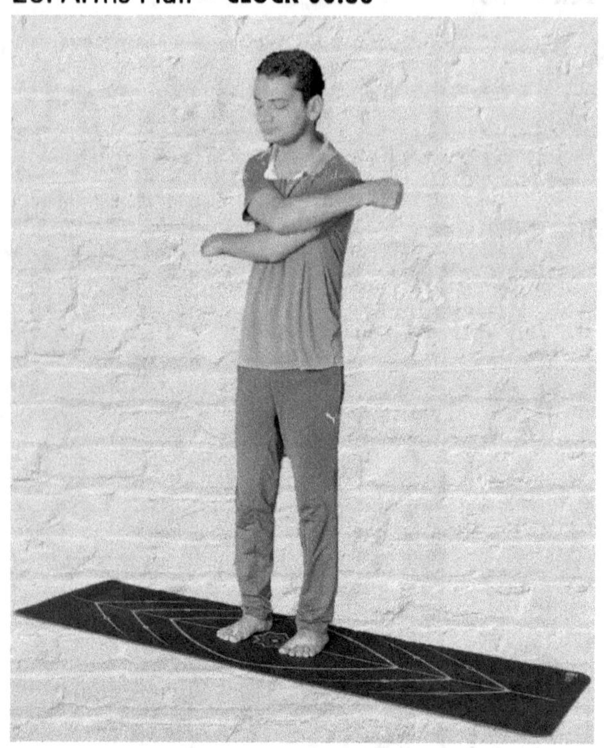

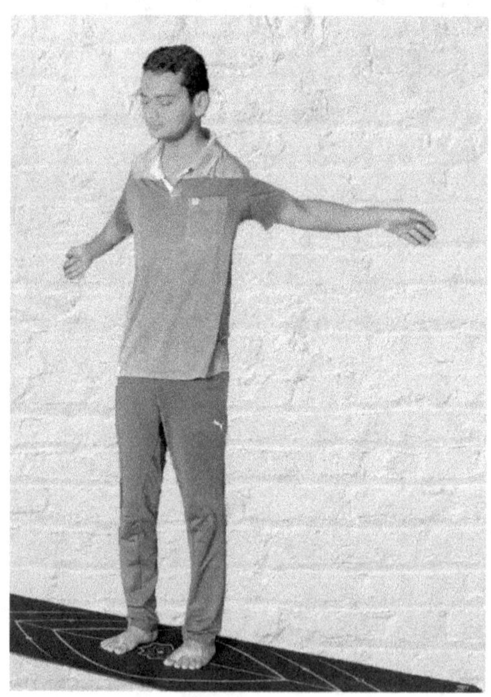

## 21. Potty Squat = **CLOCK 00:37**
malasana

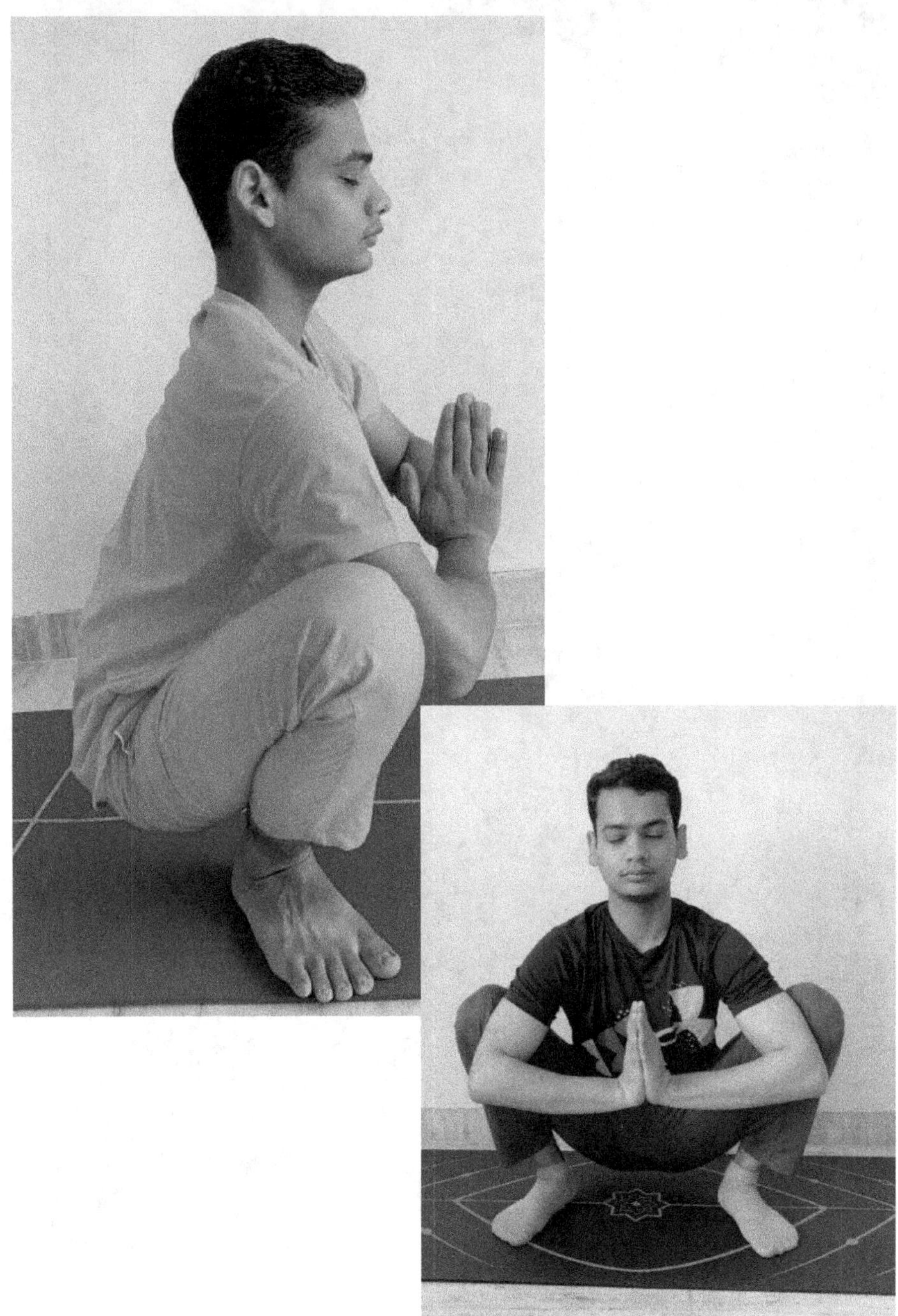

# 22. Ha! Sound Loud = **CLOCK 00:38**

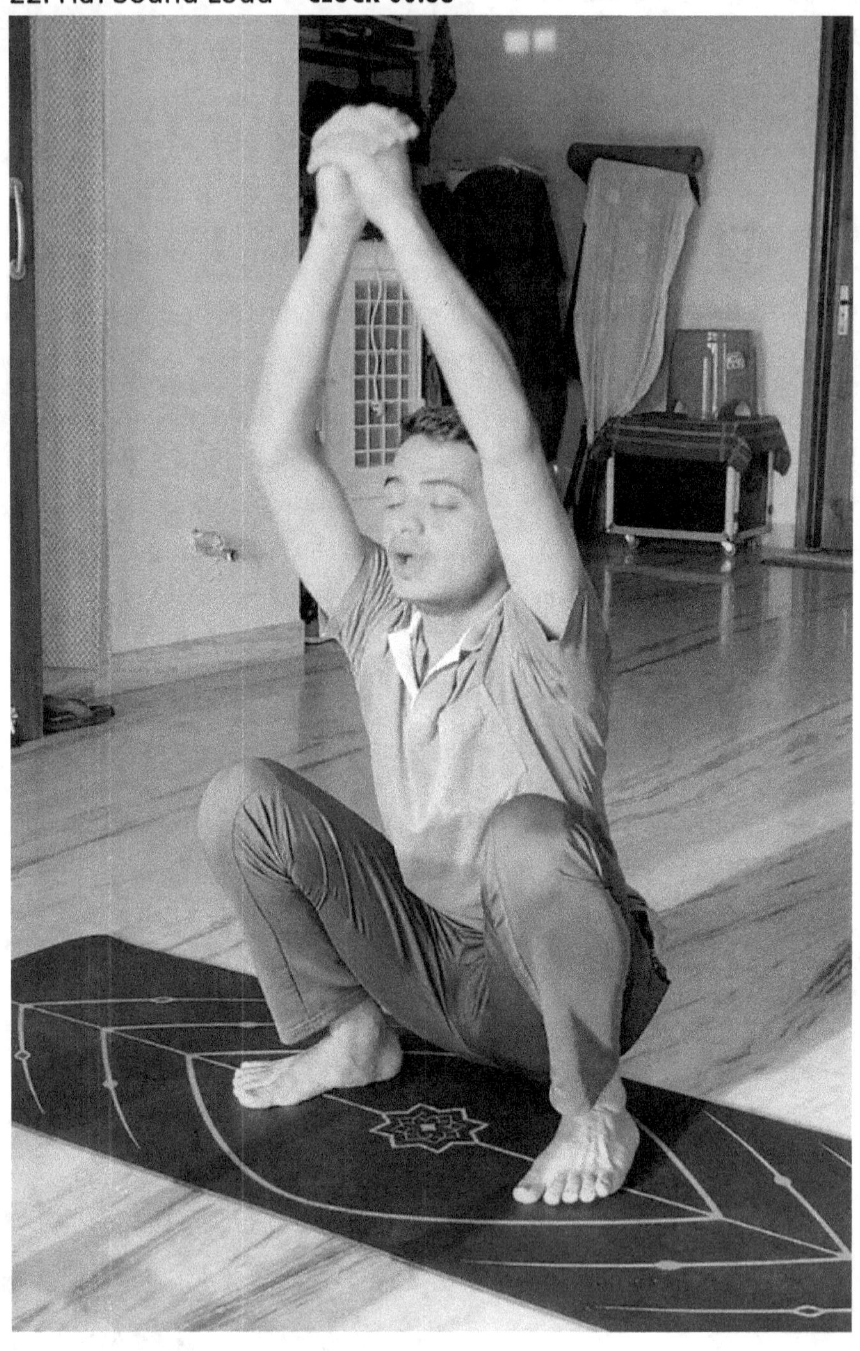

# 23. Cow Face = **CLOCK 00:39**
gomukhasana

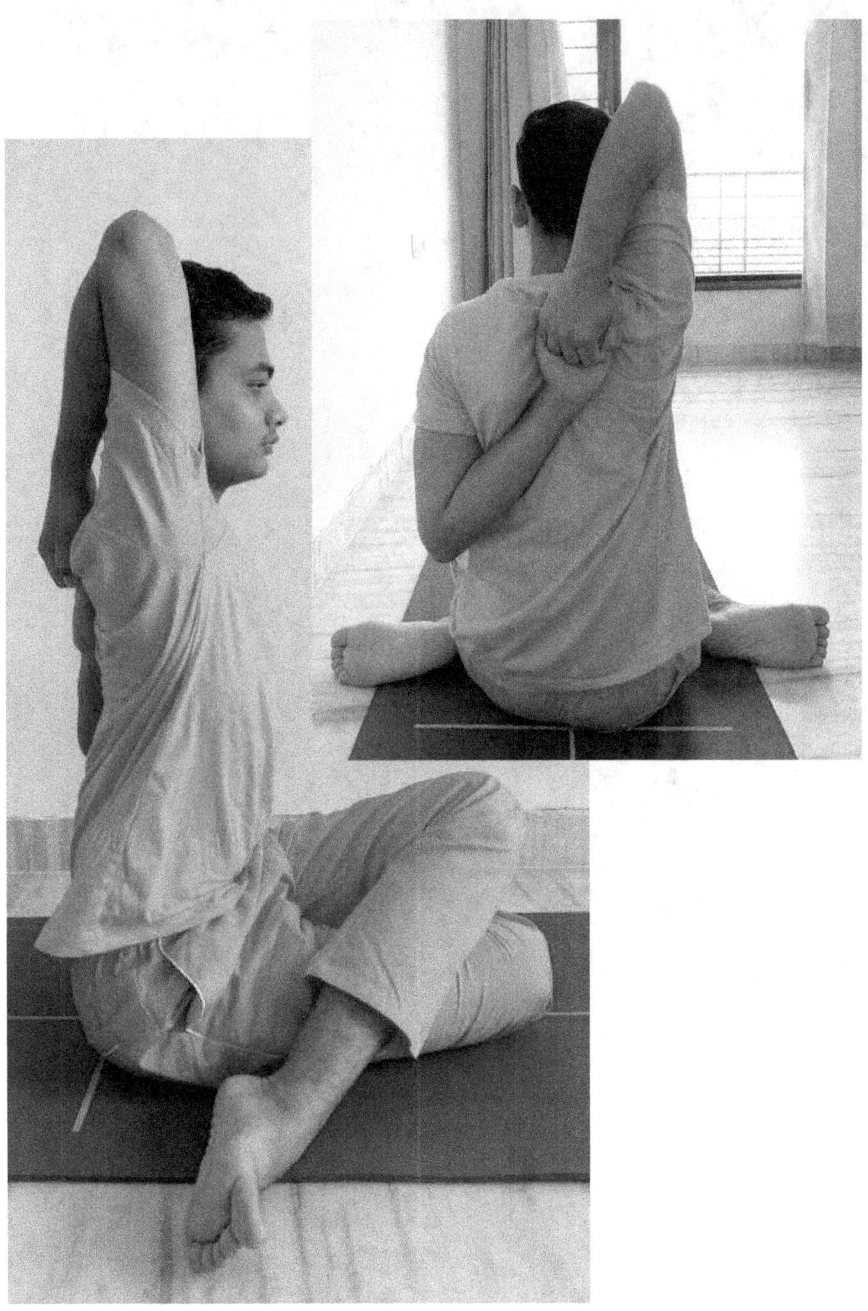

# 24. Lowered Plank = **CLOCK 00:40**
caturangasana

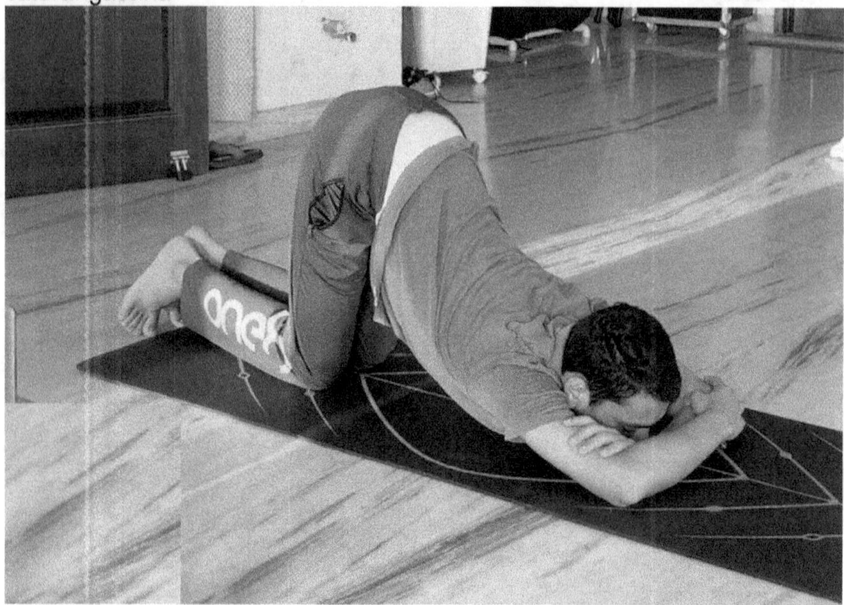

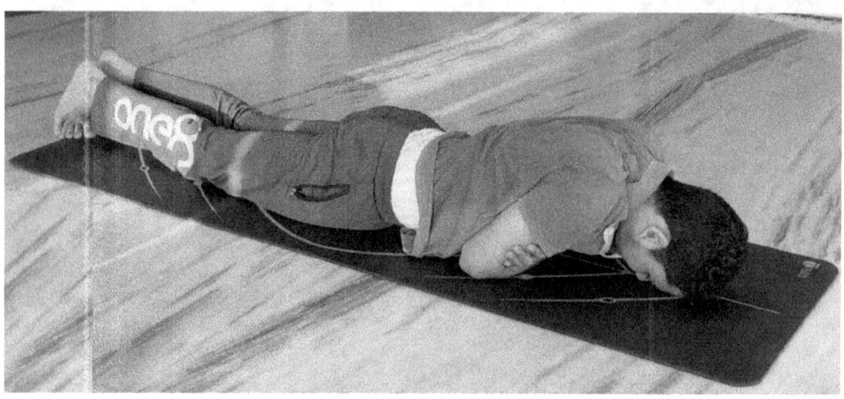

# 25. Plank = **CLOCK 00:41**
caturanga dandasana

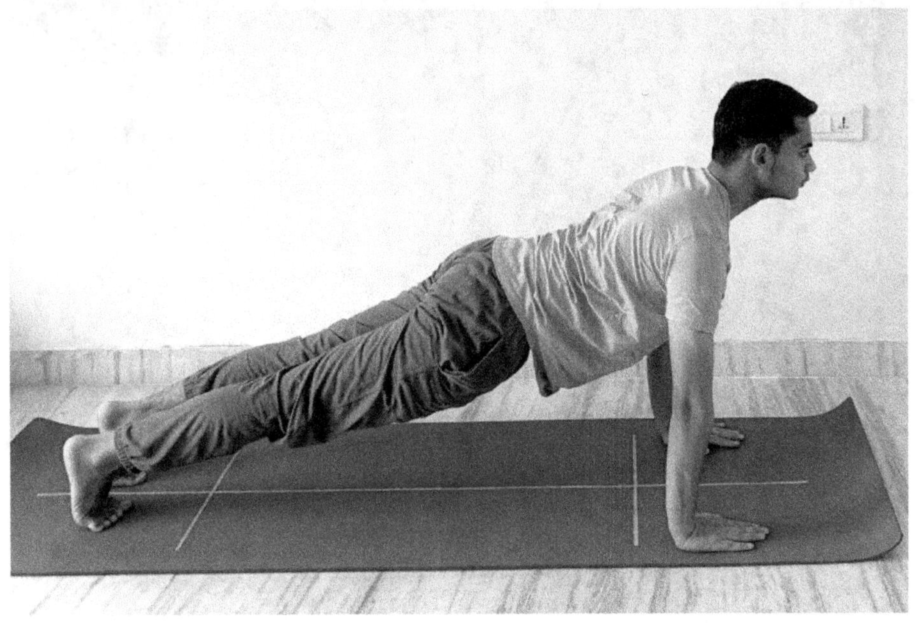

## 26. Elbow Plank = **CLOCK 00:42**
shishumar caturanga

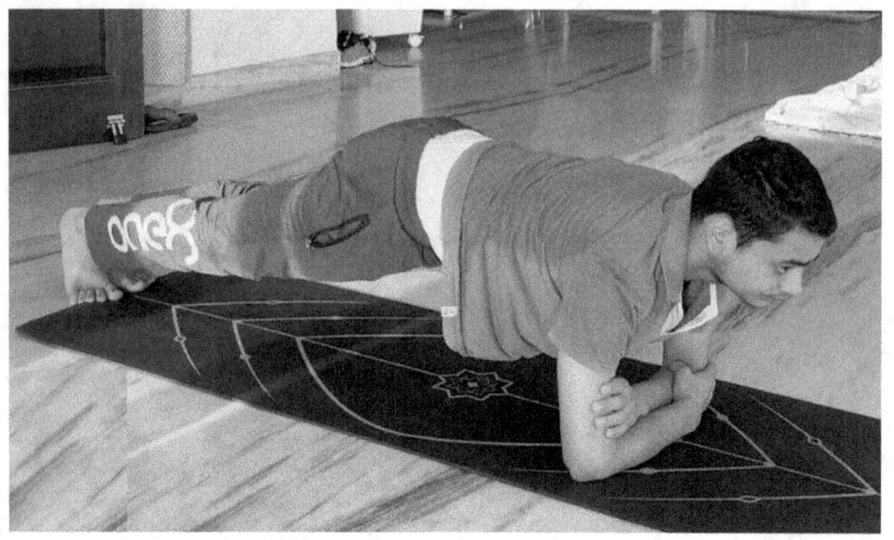

# 27. Cobra = **CLOCK 00:43** (or Sphinx)
bhujangasana

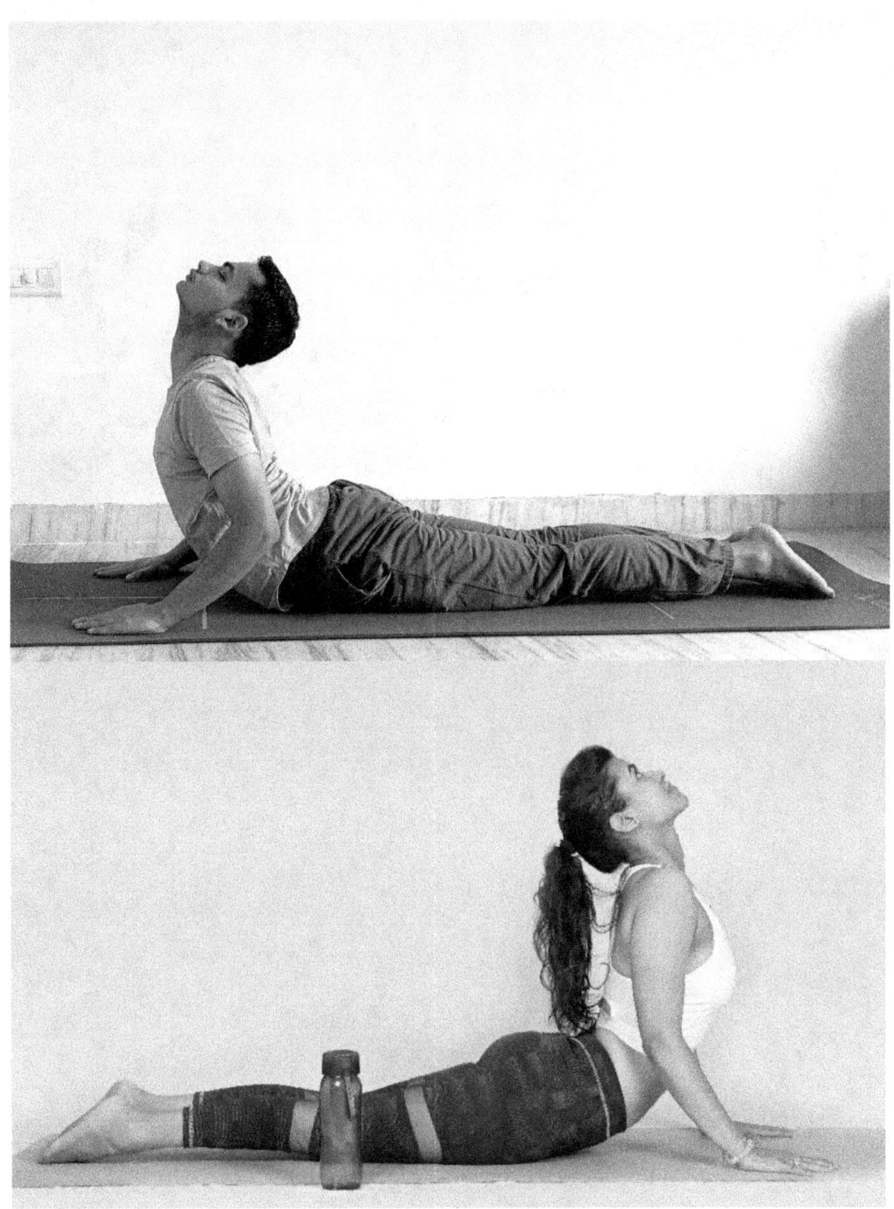

# 28. Relax Crocodile = **CLOCK 00:44**
makarasana

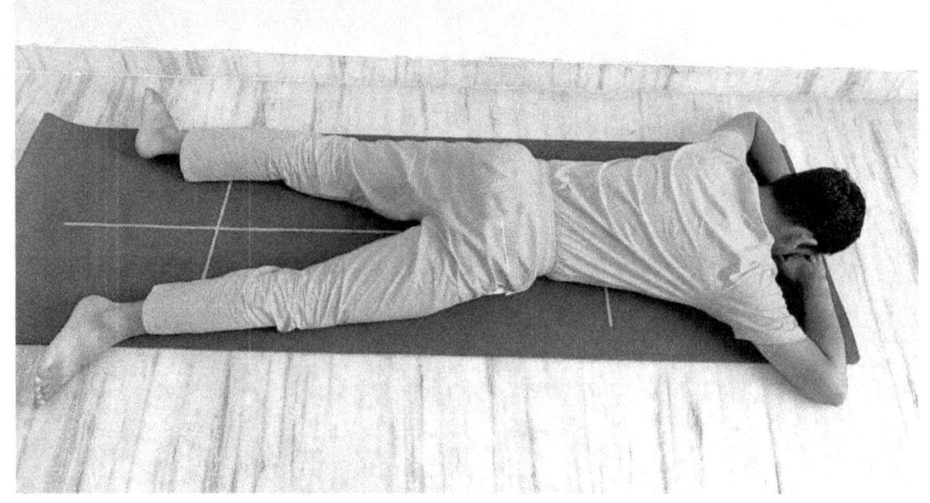

# 29. Bow = **CLOCK 00:45**
dhanurasana

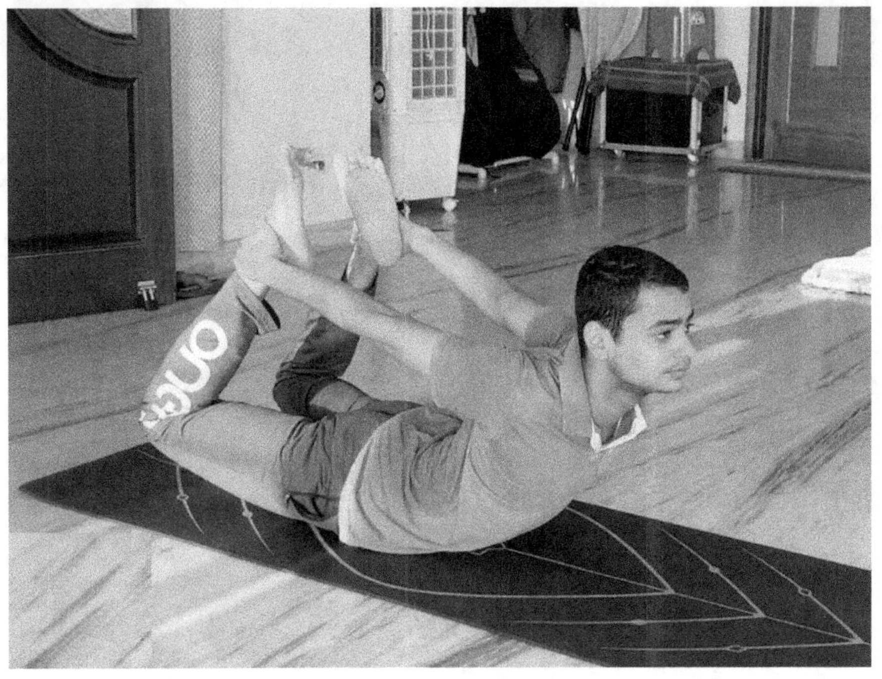

# 30. Comfortable Relax = **CLOCK 00:46**
supta vishnu asana

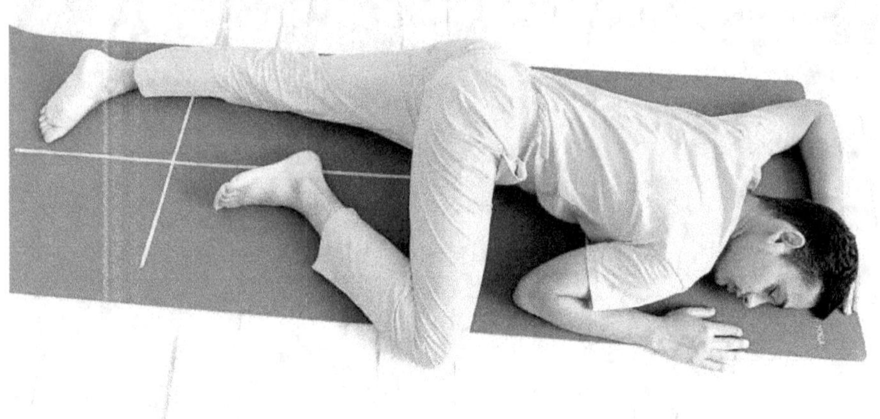

## 31. Corpse = **CLOCK 00:47**
shavasana

It is easy to think of Shavasana as of having no real importance but that is not the case. Shavasana is one of the most important asanas in Hatha Yoga.
Shavasana is mentioned in the Shiv Samhita as a meditative posture. Its effects are vast and miraculous and all cannot be listed but are certainly experienced with regular practice. Practicing

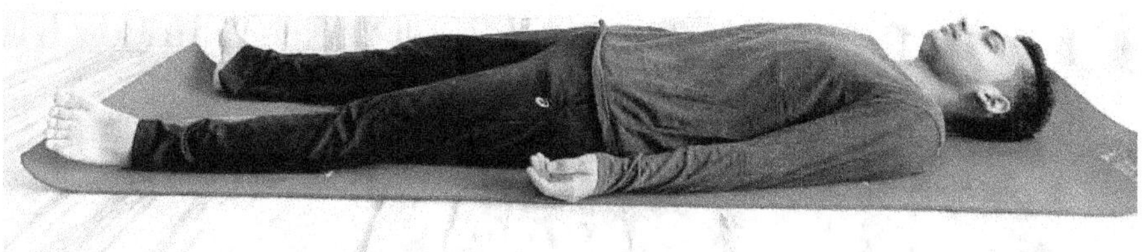

Shavasana for 8-10 minutes is absolutely essential after a workout asana session to receive the full benefit of the practice. Shavasana works on the endocrine system and makes the heart stronger.

## 32. Roll to Right side = **CLOCK 00:52**
parsva shavasana

*and then sit up. A very gentle movement.*

An essential pose after lying down asanas and sitting up. It cools the breath and relaxes the heart. It is a good practice to roll over to the right side, take a few breaths, then gently come to a sitting position using the hands and arms as support.

The heart is on the left side of the body. So when you roll to your right side, the heart remains above and that exerts less pressure on the heart.

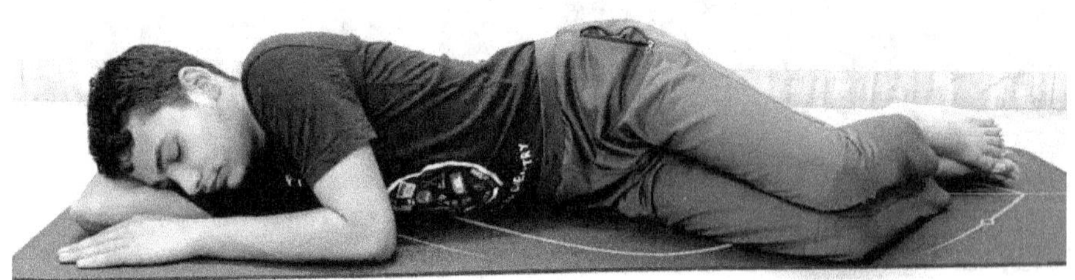

## 33. Butterfly = **CLOCK 00:53**
titli asana

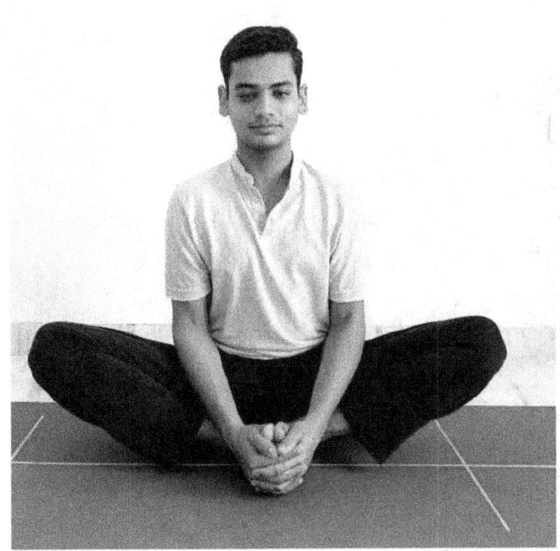

Flapping the wings, slowly at first, and then picking up speed.

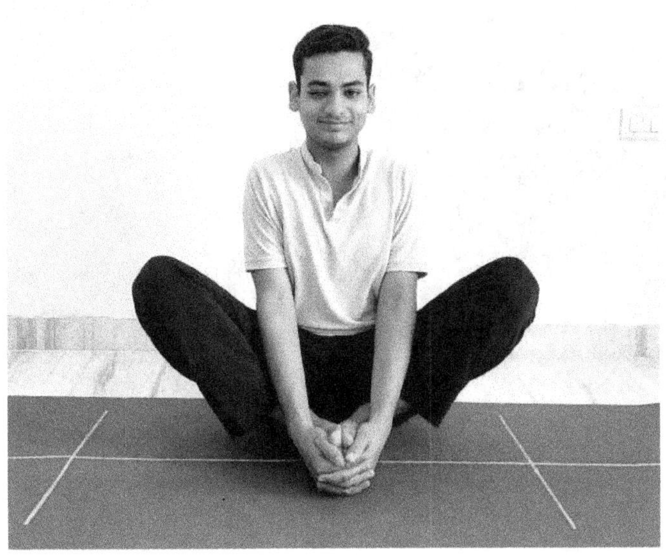

# 34. Sitting Forward Bend = **CLOCK 00:54**
paschimottanasana

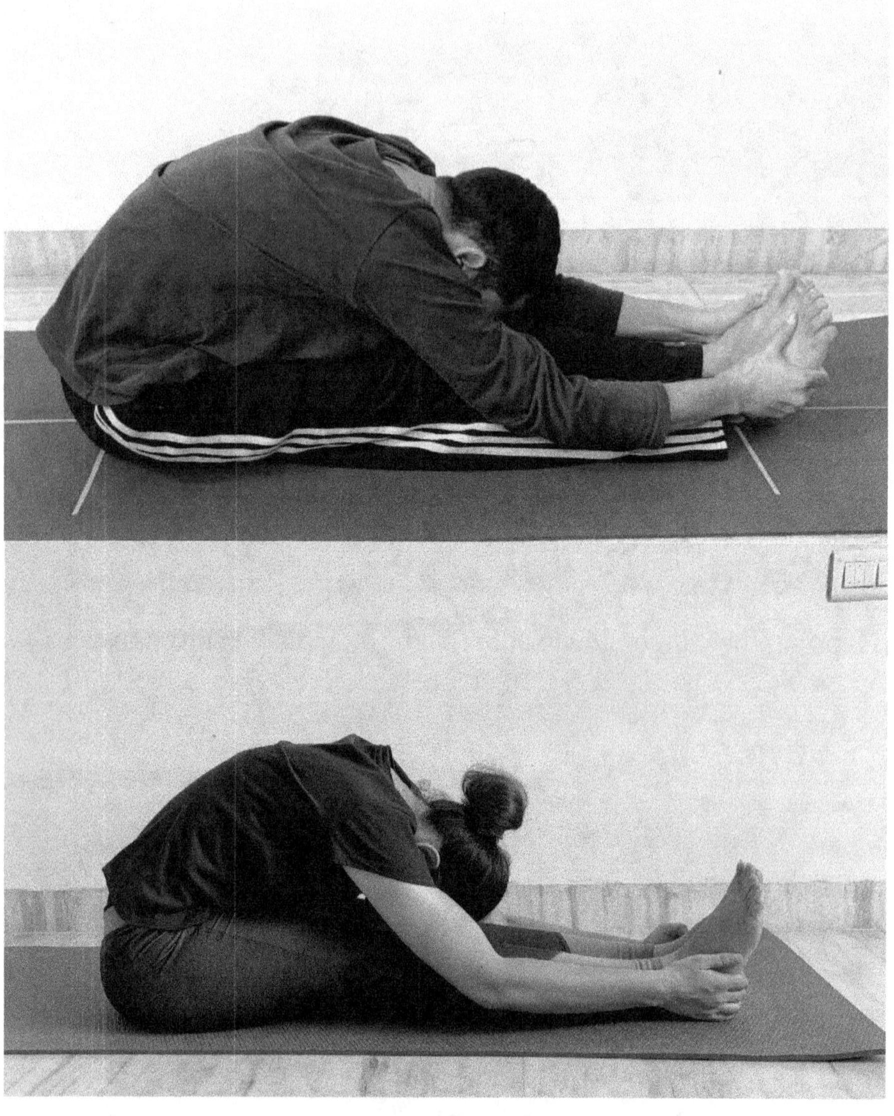

## 35. Sitting Sideways Twist = **CLOCK 00:55**
vakrasana

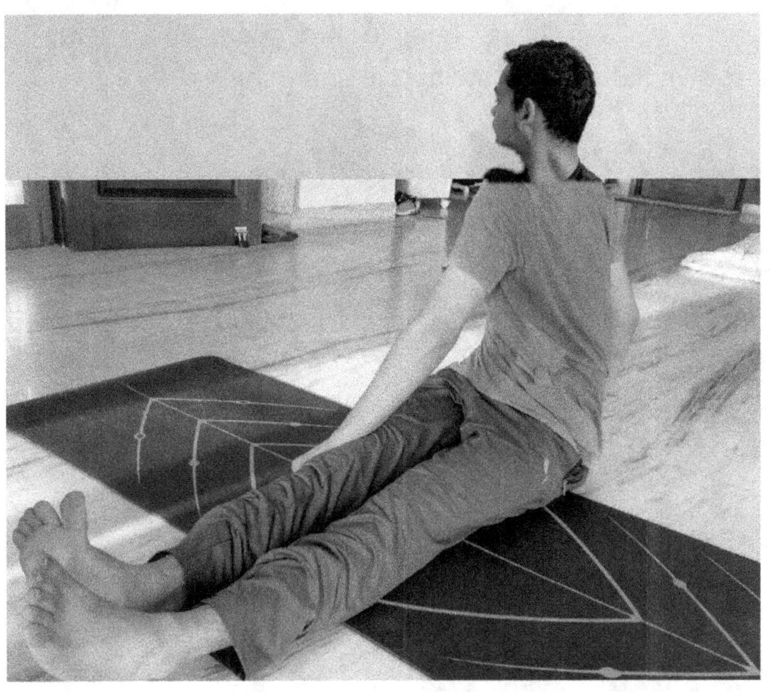

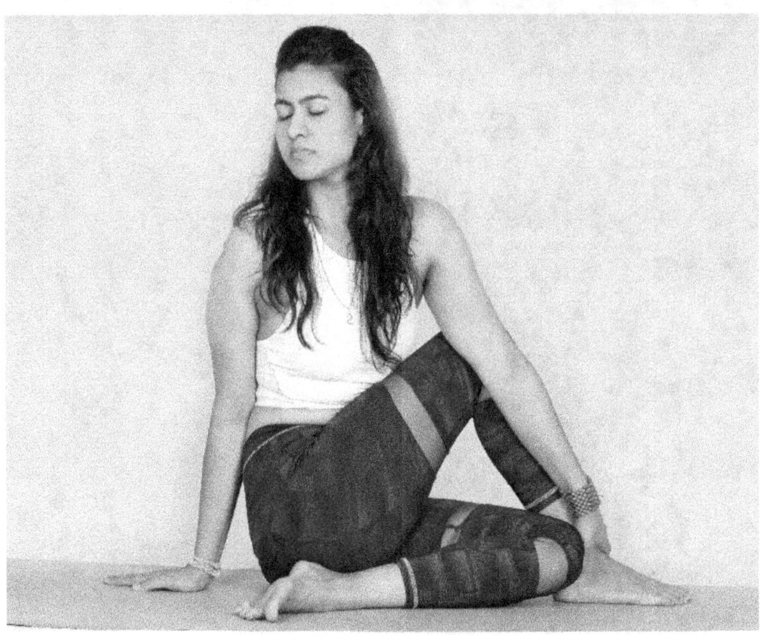

## 36. Alternate Nostril Breathing = **CLOCK 00:56**

nadi shodhan pranayama (anulom vilom pranayama)

For Pranayama, we keep the left hand in chin mudra, and use the right hand to switch the alternate nostril breathing.

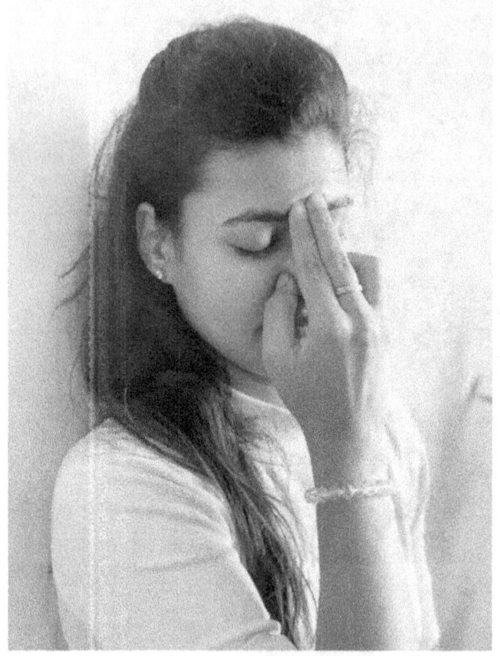

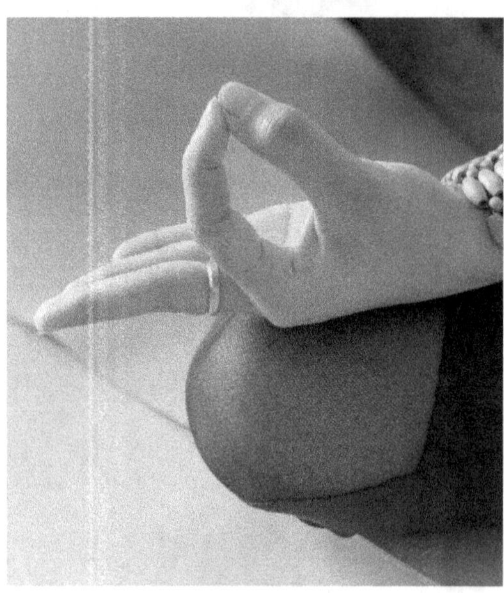

## 37. Heart Center Anahata Chakra = **CLOCK 00:58**

anahata chakra locate near thymus on sternum in chest

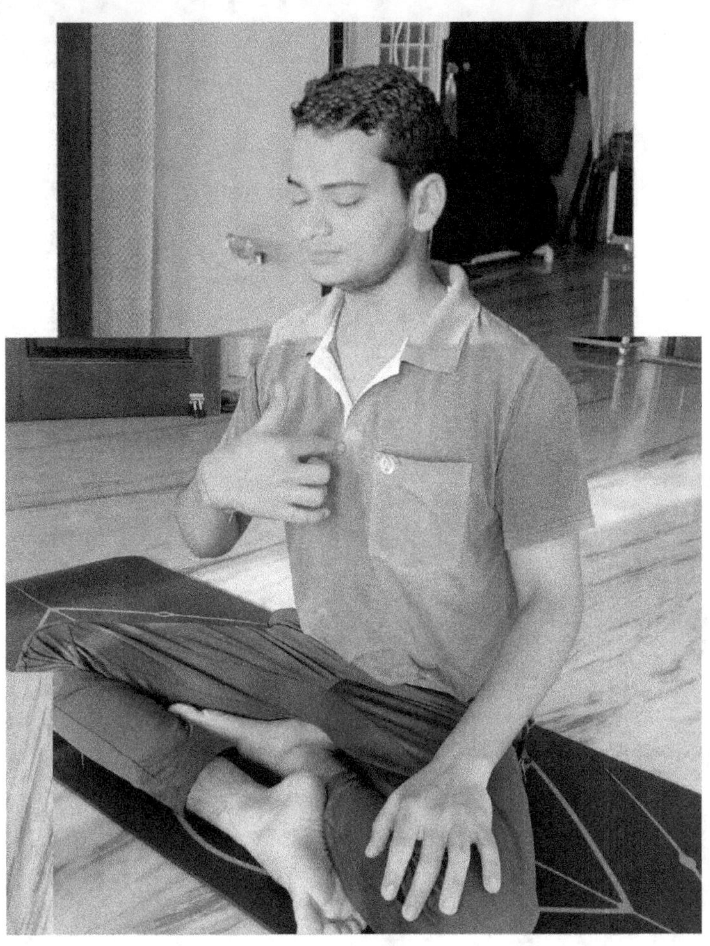

# 38. Final Meditation in Dhyana Mudra = **CLOCK 01:00**
dhyana mudra

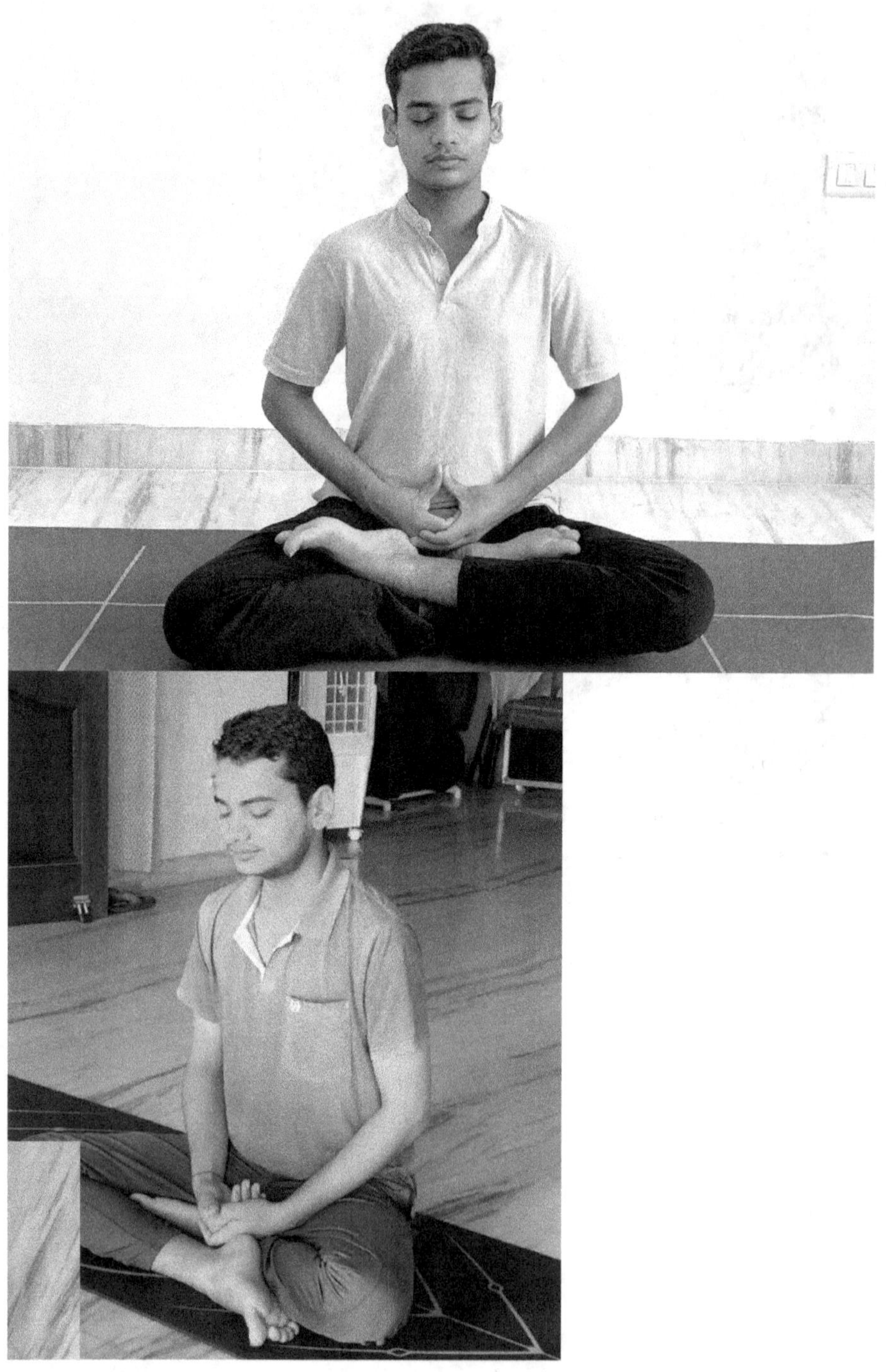

# Relaxation Poses 39

It is always necessary to relax and keep the breath normal while doing asanas. Some of the relaxation postures that are recommended for all are given here, and these can be interspersed at will during one's workout.

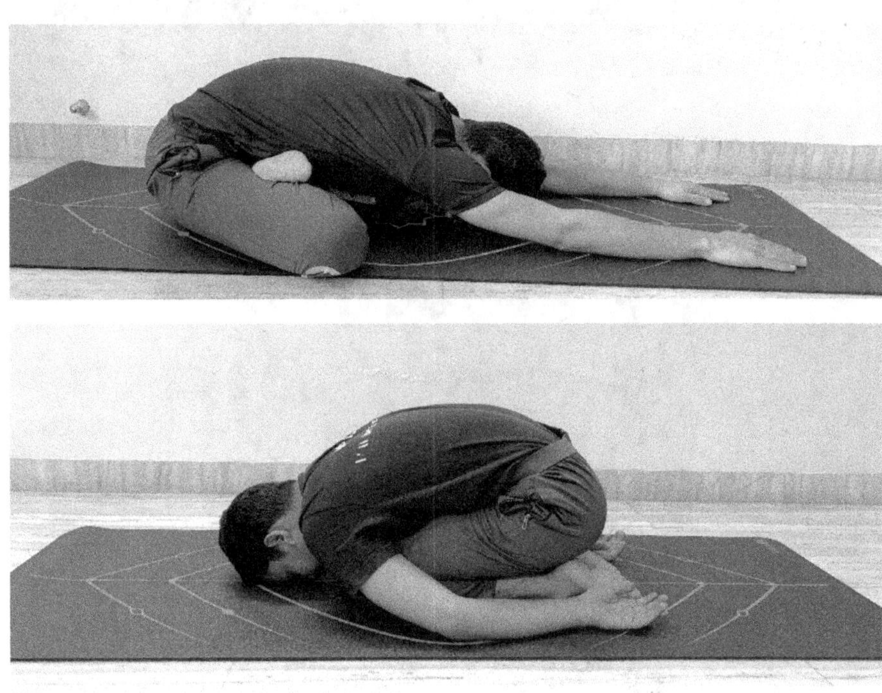

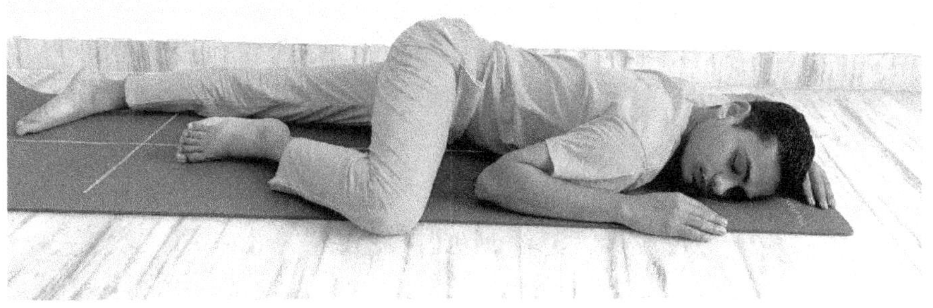

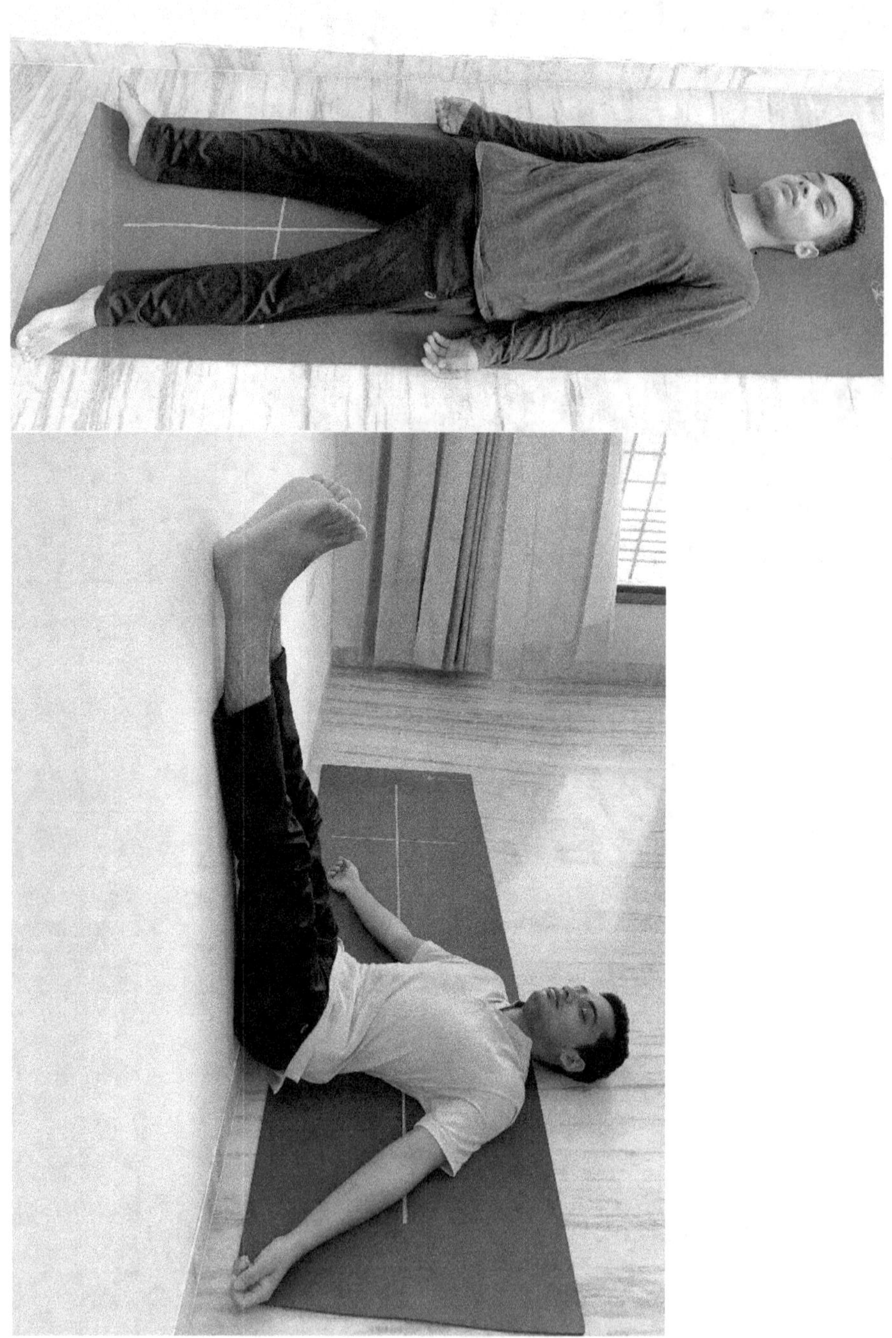

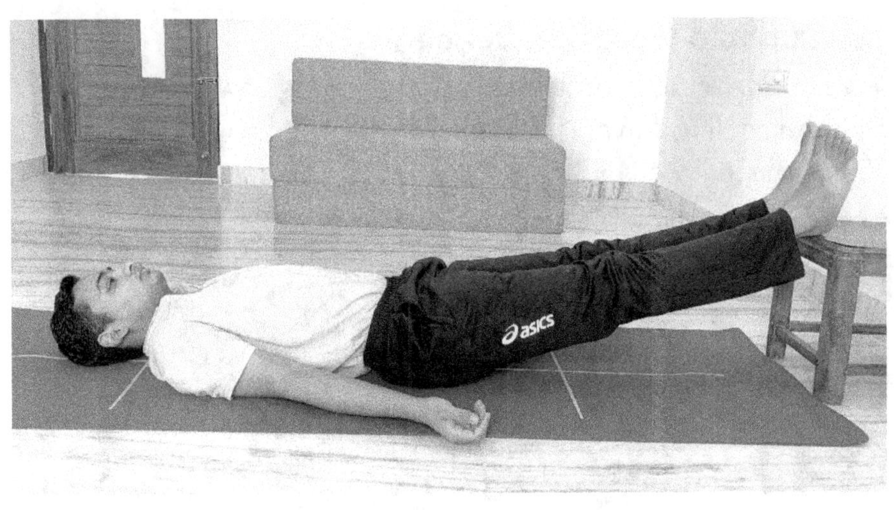

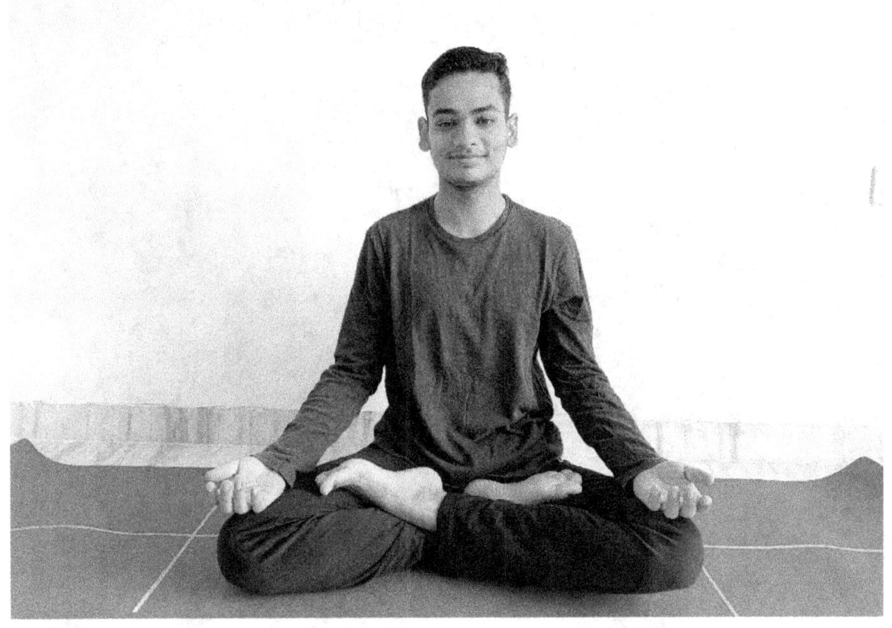

# Asana photo visual sequence

Any exercise session must begin with loosening or warming up, and end with cooling down. The standard cooling down in this case is Shavasana followed by Meditation.

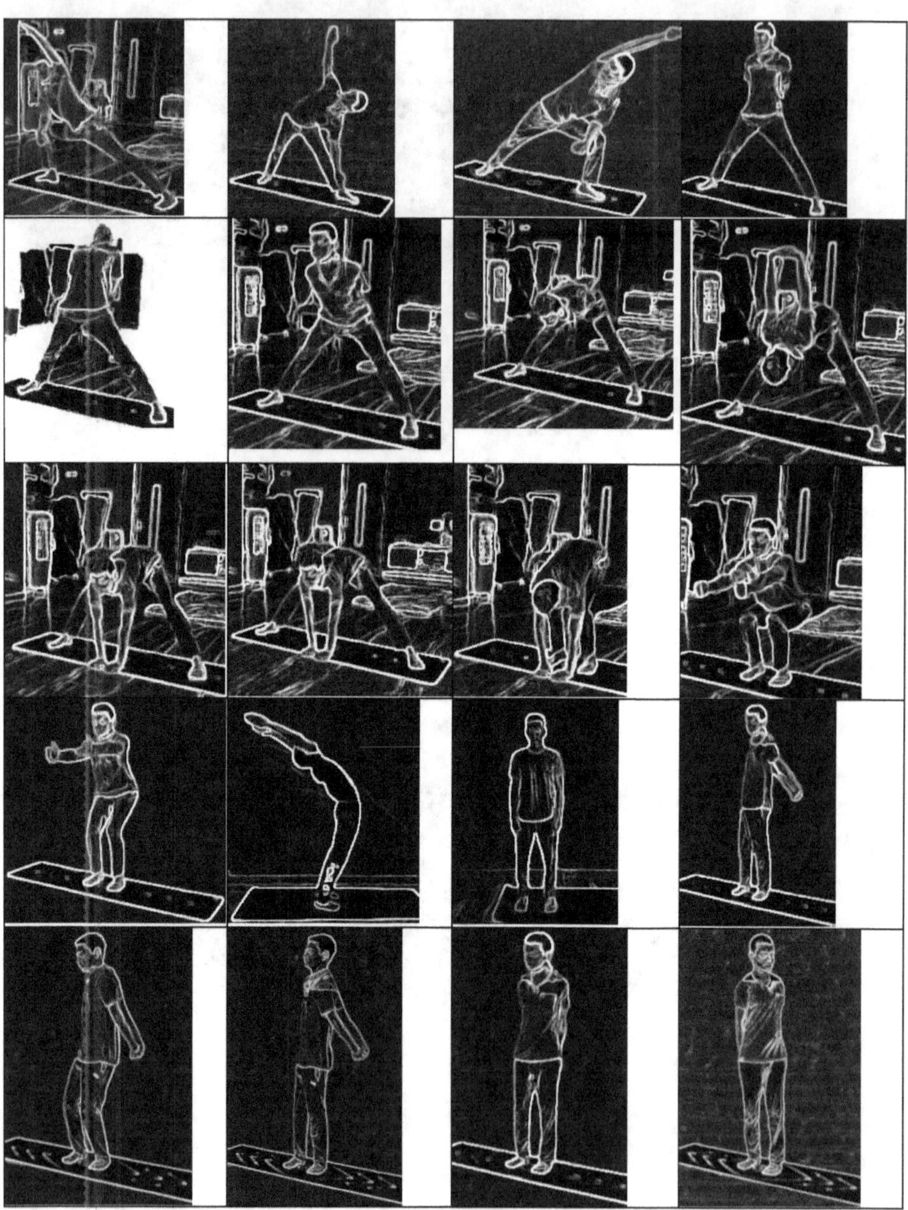

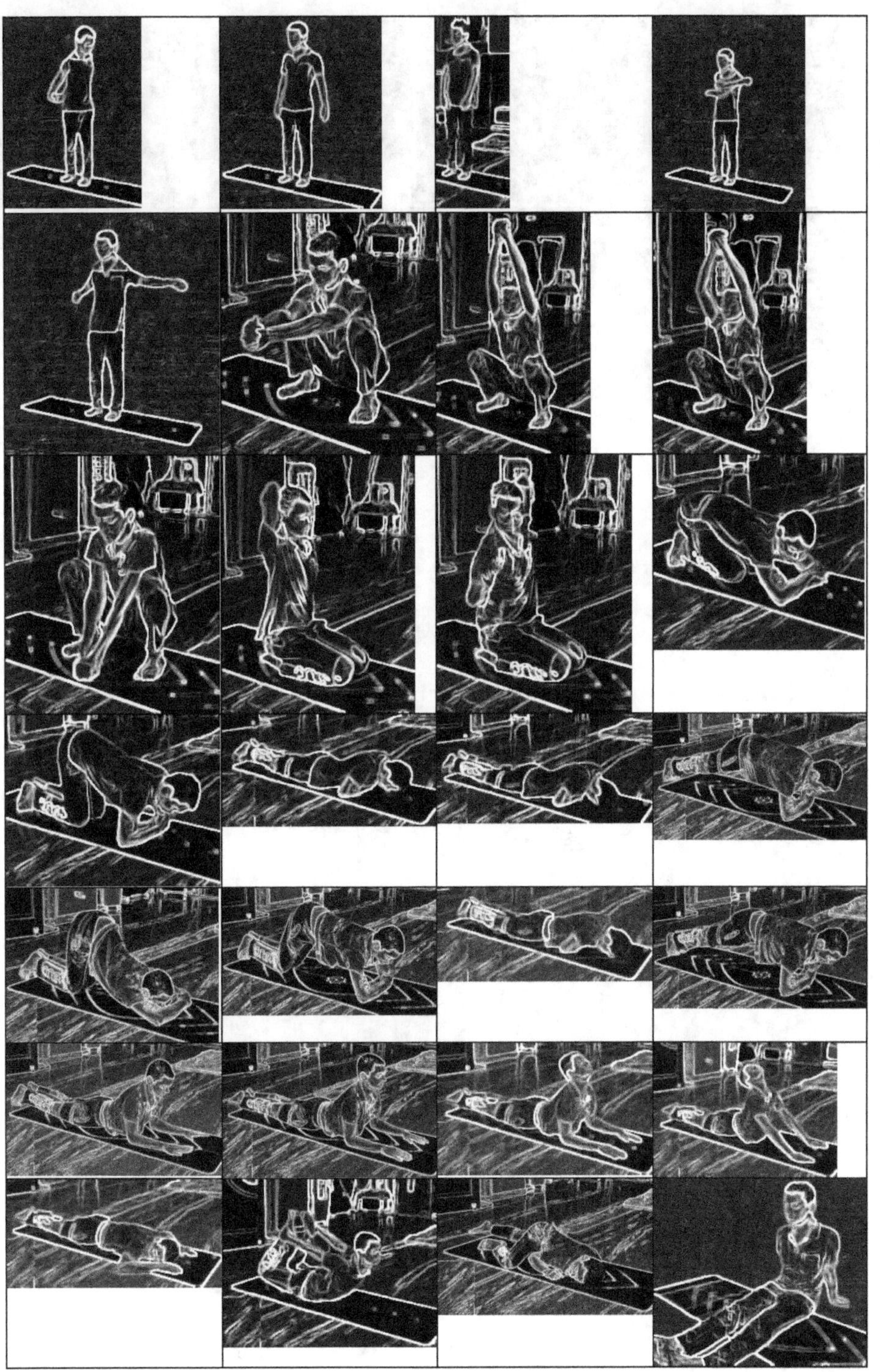

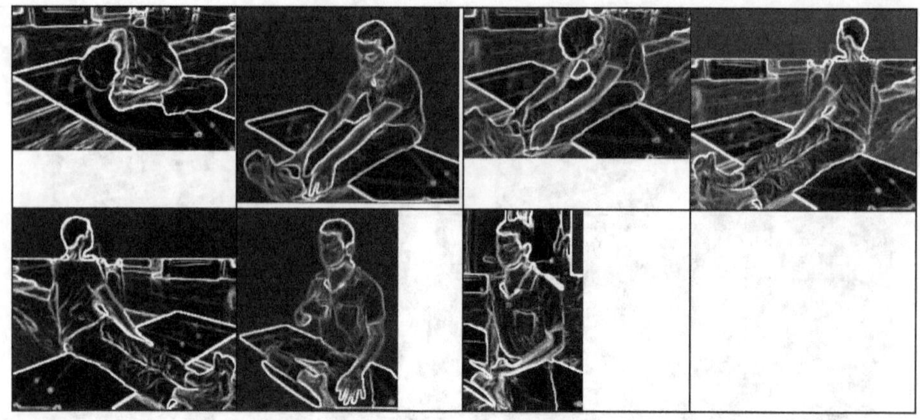

# Regular Habits

Apart from asana practice, some habits support our spirit and nurture us from a deeper plane of existence.

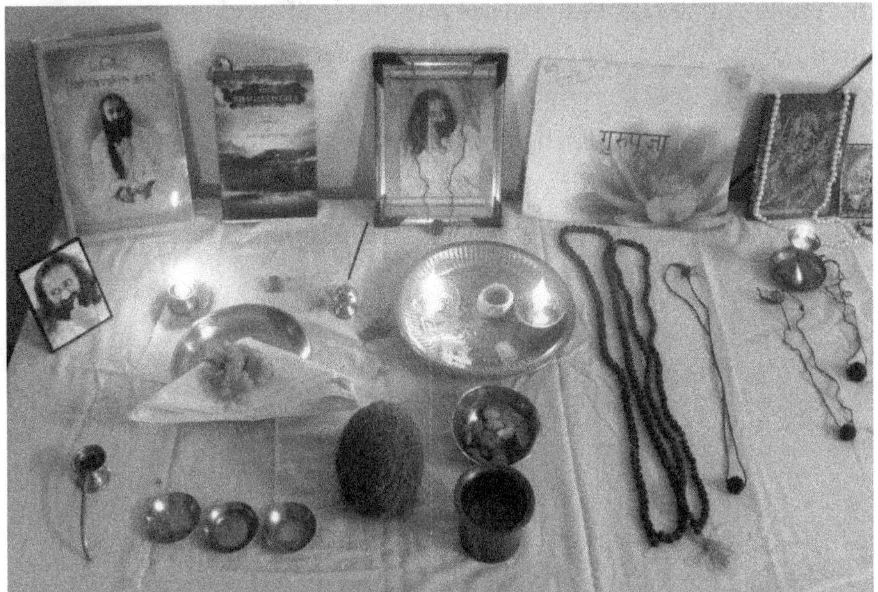

Chanting, Prayer, Lighting a Lamp, Puja Havan Satsang Aarti.

## Ayurveda

Be sure of what suits your palate, and it is safe and ecofriendly to go vegetarian. Nadi Pariksha is a safe mechanism to match our diet to our native constitution. It will prevent many ills and mood swings. And it goes without saying that locally grown fresh fruits and vegetables, and A2 cow milk products should be a diet priority. Replacing white sugar with honey, and jaggery, sea salt with rock salt, and refined oils with cold pressed mustard or groundnut oil, such culinary methods make a remarkable turnaround in overall health levels.

## Vitamins

We must supplement our diet with Sri Sri Shakti Drops and Vitamins. It is advisable to add 4 drops to a cup of water and drink daily.

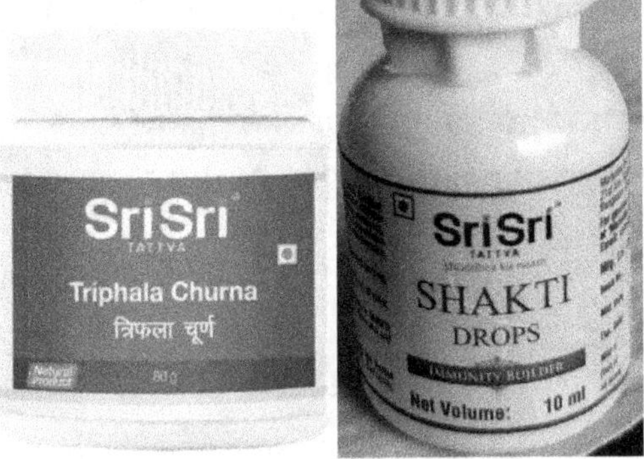

Eat a teaspoon of Triphala Churna with warm water at bedtime for a fortnight. Wash your eyes daily with Triphala water for ten days.

## Eye Care & Tooth Care

Eyes are most beautiful and need to be kept functional till a ripe old age. We can wash them with triphala water that has been strained using a fine cloth. Also, keep a tissue paper dipped in cool Rose water over the eyes and relax for a few minutes with eyes closed.

Keeping healthy teeth and gums is no longer possible by regular brushing alone due to a drastic intake of packaged and fast foods. Daily Patanjali Dant Kanti manjan is a must.

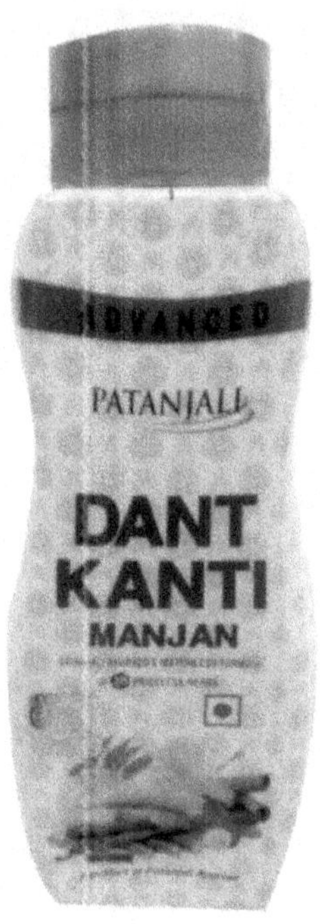

# Index of Asana

Here the alphabetical names in Sanskrit along with SNo of the Asana from Table of Contents is given.

| Asana | SNo |
| --- | --- |
| anahata chakra = heart center | 37 |
| bahu chankramana = arms flail | 20 |
| bala pada vikshepan = powerwalk | 1 |
| bandha moolbandha jalandhar = locks | 5 |
| bhitti viparita karani = legs rested | 39 |
| bhujang āsana = cobra (or sphinx pose) | 27 |
| caturanga = lowered plank | 24 |
| caturanga dandāsana = plank | 25 |
| deha chankramana = pelvic rotation | 4 |
| dhanur āsana = bow | 29 |
| dhyana mudra = palms during meditation | 38 |
| gomukhāsana = cow face | 23 |
| ha! loud sound | 22 |
| Hum! loud sound | 8 |
| hasta uttanāsana = up and back | 16 |
| bhastrika pranayama = bellows breathing | 3 |
| katichakra āsana = sideways twist | 18 |
| makarāsana = crocodile | 28 |
| malāsana = potty squat | 21 |
| nadi shodhan pranayama = alternate nostril | 36 |
| pada hastāsana = forward bend | 14 |
| padmāsana = lotus | 38 |
| parsva shavāsana = roll to right | 32 |
| paschimottanāsana = forward bend | 34 |
| pristha pranati = backbend | 13 |
| shavāsana = corpse | 31 |
| shishumar caturanga = elbow plank | 26 |
| skandha chankramana = shoulder roll | 19 |
| sukhāsana = cross-legged | 2 |
| supta vishnu āsana = comfortable relax | 30 |

tadāsana = standing tall                         17
thoppu karanam = sit-ups                         1
titli āsana = butterfly                          33
trikona āsana = triangle                         12
utkatāsana = chair                               15
vajrāsana = adamantine pose                      3, 23
vakrāsana = sitting sideways twist               35
viparit karani āsana = legs raised               39
virabhadra āsana = warrior 1                     10
virabhadra āsana = warrior 2                     11
yoga mudra = child pose                          39

A proper Yoga Mat for doing asana is a must for your practice.

# References

Ashwini Kumar Aggarwal– Yoga Science and Practice – 1$^{st}$ – 2020

Ashwini and Dipanshu – Yoga Surya Namaskar – 1$^{st}$ – 2020

Ashwini and Dipanshu – Gheranda Samhita the foundation of Modern Yoga – 1$^{st}$ 2020

Ashwini and Dipanshu – 84 Yoga Asanas Fitness Postures – 1$^{st}$ – 2021

Devotees of Sri Sri Ravi Shankar Ashram, Punjab.

## Epilogue

One hour a day spent towards achieving and maintaining this lifestyle is an hour well spent. Do not stretch yourself to accommodate an entire hour. The principle of the book is that if you can practice some Yoga for even as less as 10-15 minutes at a time – realign your spine, get the blood flowing, and keep the joints active – you will see a major change in the quality of physical, mental and emotional health.

सर्वे भवन्तु सुखिनः । सर्वे सन्तु निरामयाः ।

सर्वे भद्राणि पश्यन्तु । मा कश्चिद् दुःख भाग् भवेत् ॥

ॐ शान्तिः शान्तिः शान्तिः ॥

When faith has blossomed in life, Every step is led by the Divine.

Sri Sri Ravi Shankar

**Om Namah Shivaya**

जय गुरुदेव